The Basic Approach to SOT
Category I, II and III

Dr. Bruce Vaughan

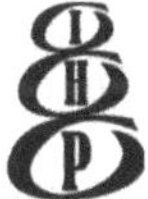

INTERNATIONAL HEALTH PUBLISHING
www.InternationalHealthPublishing.com

Carrollton, Texas, USA

INTERNATIONAL HEALTH PUBLISHING
February 22, 2008
Publishing Group Affirming Truth & Innate Wisdom

First International Health Publishing trade paperback edition December 2010

For information about special discounts for bulk purchase, please contact International Health Publishing at writer@InternationalHealthPublishing.com.

International Health Publishing can bring authors to your live events. For more information or to book an event, contact writer@InternationalHealthPublishing.com or for more information visit our website: www.InternationalHealthPublishing.com.

The Basic Approach to SOT, Category I, II and III
Dr. Bruce Vaughan
www.brucevaughan.com

ISBN-13 978-0-9818353-6-5
ISBN-10 0-9818353-6-8

Library of Congress Control Number: 2010937196

SAN 856-6925

Manufactured in the United States of America, and printed on the finest
100% postconsumer-waste recycled paper

10 9 8 7 6 5 4 3 2 1

Books by the same author:

Rabid Dogs In The East
Brazilian Saddle Sores
Regenesis
A Matter of Face

www.brucevaughan.com

Author's Note

This book is the result of several years of self study of the works of Dr. Major Bertrand De Jarnette, coupled with 44-years of chiropractic practice. Many notable SOT instructors and practitioners have contributed to my knowledge of SOT and have therefore, unknowingly, contributed to this book. This book is not intended to replace the very valuable hands-on training offered by the various SOT organizations around the world. Instead, it is meant for the senior student or DC interested in this amazing approach to chiropractic called Sacro Occipital Technic (SOT).

With this book, the student or doctor of SOT gains an understanding of the analysis and treatment protocols that have been so successful in helping patients through difficult times and painful episodes of spinal origin. It is by no means an exhaustive study, as there is so much more to SOT; but it is a start.

SOT goes beyond mere pain relief. It looks to the integrity and balance of the entire spine, corrects the cause of the imbalance as well as the myriad of secondary problems that can arise. Once you have become involved in this amazing approach you will find that it will answer those important questions:

What is the cause of the patients' problem?
What to do today?
What not to do?
When is it 'fixed'?

If this book arouses your interest in SOT, learn what you can from it and then attend the multitude of seminars available through the various SOT organisations around the world.

Bruce Vaughan

Foreword

I am honored to write the foreword for this wonderful book, *The Basic Approach to SOT, Category I, II, and III.* Having had the opportunity to meet with Dr. Bruce Vaughan and discuss sacro-occipital technique (SOT) with him in depth, it was wonderful to see his dedication and desire to share the depth of his understanding of this method of chiropractic developed by Major Bertrand DeJarnette, DO, DC called SOT.

Dr. Vaughan incorporates his years of clinical expertise with his understanding of SOT enhanced by his graphic artist skills to present representative pictorials of SOT analysis and treatment. His insight into sharing some novel methods of utilizing SOT principles will help both students learning SOT and doctors long in SOT practice.

He utilizes his literary skills also to present an easy to read and follow step by step method of learning how to analyze, diagnose and treat the three SOT categories developed by Dr. DeJarnette.

While it is easy to make SOT categories complicated and hard to learn, the real skill that Dr. Vaughan has perfected is a manner of presenting information that is easily digested and assimilated.

Charles Blum, DC
Santa Monica, California 90405

Contents

The Basic Approach to SOT
Category I, II and III

Dr. Bruce Vaughan

Introduction

The adaptation to the erect stance of man put a great burden of responsibility on the structures that make up the pelvic girdle. The pelvis is the foundation for the musculo-skeletal structures both above and below it. A sound base gives rise to a sound structure, whereas an unsound or distorted base cannot help but lead to faulty structure and thence faulty function.

The Sacro-iliac articulations bear the full-weight of the erect human torso without the assistance of muscular support. The SI Joint is by no means the solid immovable bonding that it was held out to be by so many medical pundits. It is an immensely strong union that supports the body, however it does allow for a variety of movements for a variety of reasons.

Movements of the Sacro-iliac Joint, barely measurable though they may be, are essential for the well being as well as the mobility and locomotion of man.

The skull contains the Brain and the spine contains the Spinal Cord, both of which are bathed in and nurtured by Cerebro-Spinal Fluid (CSF). The CSF is contained within the Dura Mater extending from the Skull to the Sacrum. Circulation of the CSF from the Skull ot the Spine relies on movement of the bones of the skull and the Sacrum. This movement, which usually coincides with the respiratory cycle, alternately lengthens and shortens the spine. This essentially mechanism, called the PRIMARY RESPIRATORY MECHANISM, will be explained in detail later. In order to understand the mechanism of pelvic movement, it is essential to study the Sacro-Iliac Joint.

The SI Joint is mostly a dry hyaline interosseous cartilage suspending the Sacrum between the Ilia. There is a smaller area of the articulation that is synovial. This wet synovial diarthrodial articulation is **BOOT shaped**, or if you prefer it, L-shaped, with a smooth surface where the movement takes place. There are no voluntary muscles that cross the Sacra-iliac Joints, although a strong system of interosseous ligaments limit the amount of movement as well as give the strength required to support body weight.

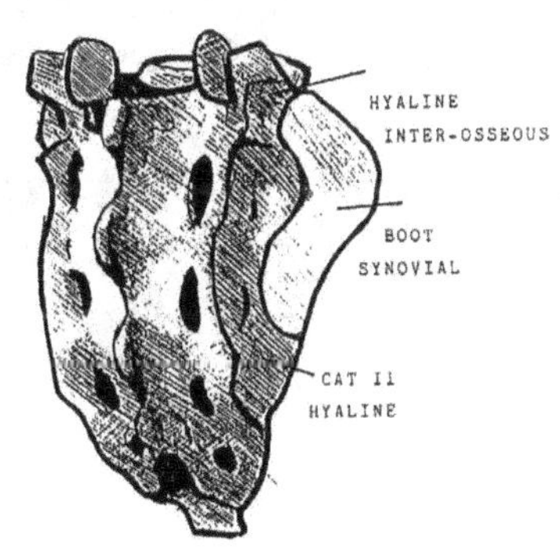

INTRODUCTION

Movement of the Pelvis is the result of leg and/or torso movement; and the Sacrum, suspended as it is between the two Ilia, absorbs and redirects movement to allow balance and stability. It is like the give and take in the framework of a wooden ship.

THE AXES OF SACRAL MOTION

The CSF pump (BOOT) action is a NODDING movement whose axis is the **AXIAL LIGAMENT,** which lies posterior to the interosseous hyaline cartilage adjacent to the postero-lateral union of S1/S2.

A line connecting the two Axial Ligaments would hypothetically pass through, or close to the point where the DURA MATER attaches to the body of S2.

R	Respiratory
M	Mean Transverse
ST	Superior Transverse
IT	Inferior Transverse
O	Oblique
V	Verticle

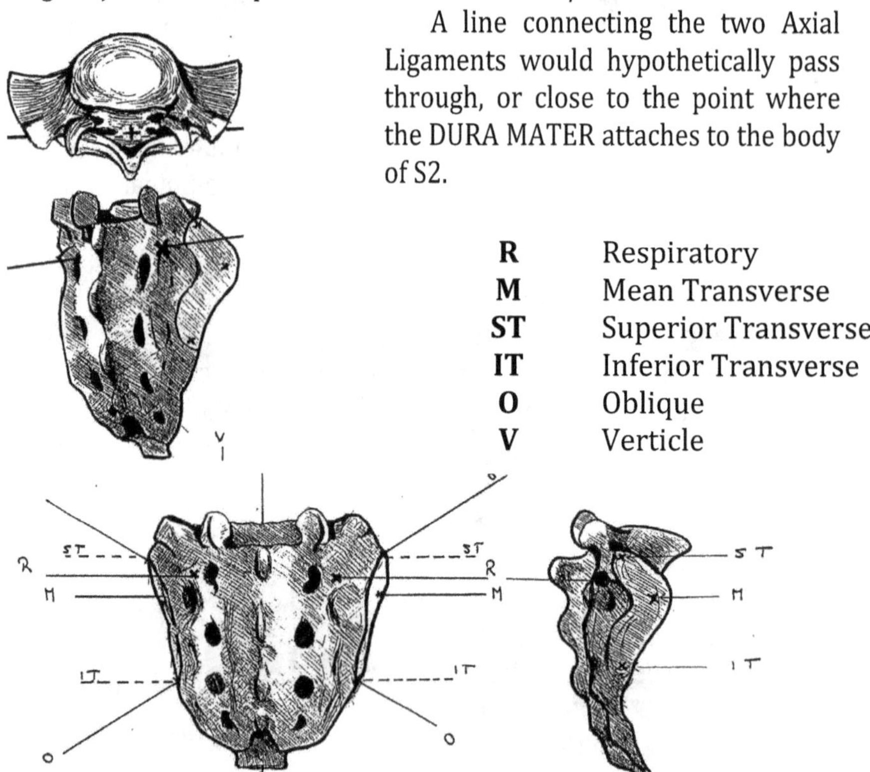

The movement of the SI Joint during walking and bending also takes place at the synovial joint, but with different axes. There are six axes illustrated: three transverse, two obliques and one verticle.

The essential connection between the occiput and the Sacrum is through the **DURA MATER,** the tough protective membrane that envelops the brain and the spinal cord. As the DURA MATER leaves the skull, it is attached to the foramen magnum and the bodies of the Axis and C3 vertebrae. There is no further connection of the DURA MATER throughout the length of the spine until it reaches the Sacrum, where it attaches to the body of S2 and then becomes the **FILUM TERMINALE**.

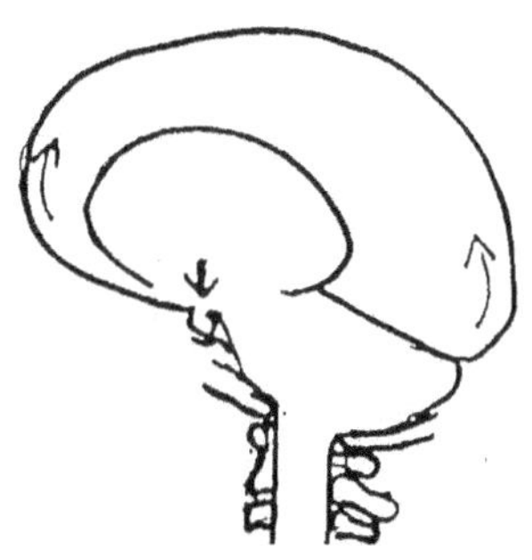

There is however, attachment of the DURA MATER at the segmental level as the nerve root exits the intervertebral foramen. The NODDING or FLEXION/ EXTENSION movement stretches and shortens the DURA MATER, enhancing circulation of the **CEREBRAL SPINAL FLUID** (CSF) acting as a form of bellows.

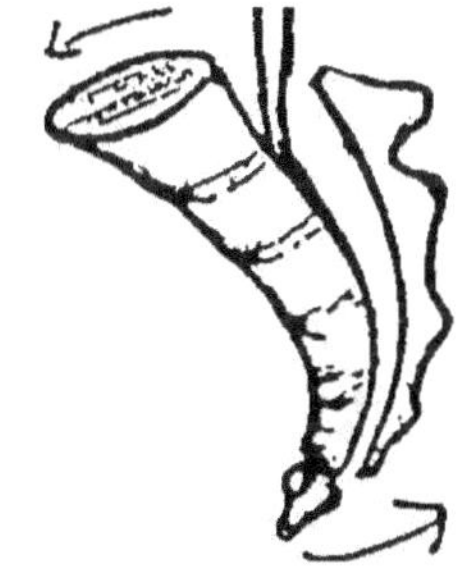

When we breathe, our lungs expand and air fills up the space created. The skull expands with inhalation (Sacral EXTENSION), and the skull contracts on exhalation (Sacral FLEXION). With the help of the spinal concert of motion, the breath and Sacral pumping cause an up-and-down flow of the CSF.

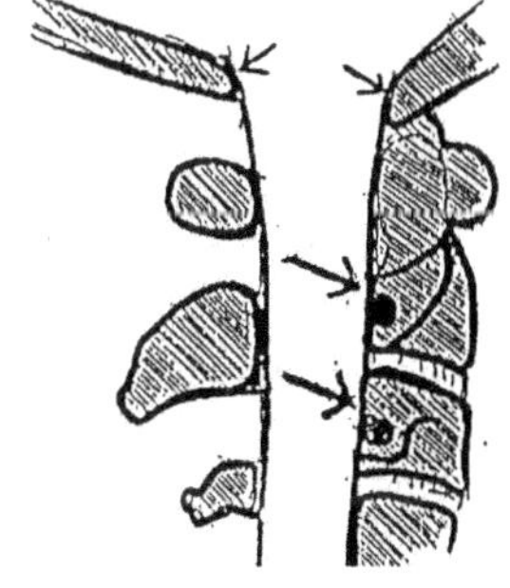

The arrows show the points of DURAL attachment at the Foramen Magnum, the bodies of the Axis and C3. The next point of attachment is at the level of S2. Other attachments have been reported to muscles and ligaments in the region. For further reading on this subject, please reference Appendix I – Dural Connections (p. 107).

The Occiput and Sacrum nod in usison during respiration through

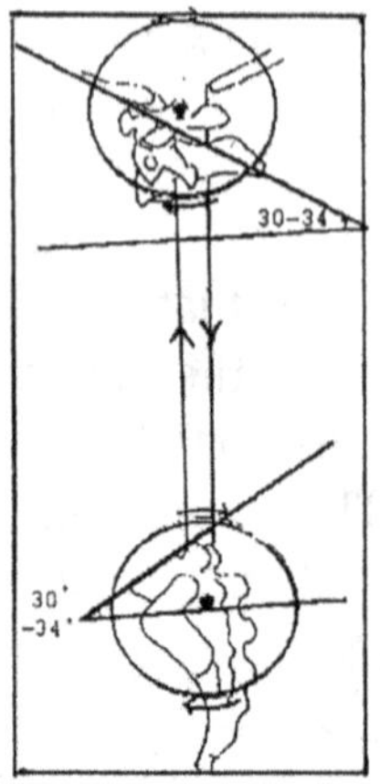

their DURA MATER connection. In the erect person, ideally the base of the Sacrum should be set at an angle of 30° - 34° in relation to the floor. This is also true of the spheno-basal line of the skull.

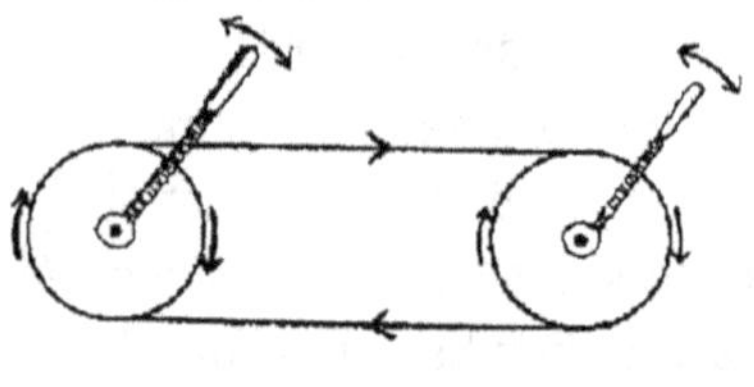

To illustrate this Sacro-occipital connection, consider the mechanism of a remote control lever worked by a pulley. When the lever is pushed forward the gear at the other end of the pulley will also move forward. With this example, if the lever is stuck then the gear mechanism will also be stuck and vice versa. The Sacral movement is equally dependent on Occipital movement and vice versa.

THE FIRST BREATH THAT KICK-STARTS THE MECHANISM

When a child is born and takes their first breath of life, the **NORMAL PHYSIOLOGICAL CATEGORY I** is set into motion. Barring incidents or accidents, that baby will spend a long and fruitful life as a normal PHYSIOLOGICAL CAT I and the mechanism will close down as the last breath of life is exhaled.

CATEGORY I

When the **BOOT** mechanism becomes impaired by whatever means, there is a torque-locking action along one of the Oblique Axes, and the Sacral part of the respiratory mechanism can no longer function. A complex distortion can then ensue, creating **Dural Torque**. This is the **PATHOLOGICAL CAT I**, and is the start of a *sick* patient.

CATEGORY II

When there is sufficient stress or trauma exerted on the pelvis, the dry hyaline cartilage that binds the Sacro-iliac articulation becomes wet, weakened or damaged, and the weight-bearing mechanism becomes unstable. Because the pelvis is the origin for the main muscles supporting and moving both the trunk and the legs, the unstable weight-bearing mechanism can have far reaching consequences.

There are three sub-classifications of the CAT II:

Traumatic Separation is a rare but severe major breakdown in the weight bearing mechanism with actual separation.

Sprain is a severe insult to the weight bearing mechanism, short of separation.

Strain is usually a chronic structure overload, which can go undetected but be responsible for more far reaching symptoms, including the TMJ problem.

CATEGORY III

The continued presence of a **PATHOLOGICAL CAT I** or a **CAT II** can lead to stress in the Lumbar spine and resultant wear with eventual deterioration of one or more discs. All too often this leads to neurological impairment and the classic sciatica. For an SOT practitioner, this is the **CAT III problem**.

There are a number of variations of the **CAT III complex,** depending on whether there is Annulus Compression, Nucleus Bulge, Rotation or Tippage. Sacral Tippage and Piriformis or Psoas weakness also enter into the equation. These variations will be dealt with during the discussions of CAT III correction.

THE AIM OF SOT CORRECTION

The most important element to understand is that the aim of any SOT procedure is to restore the sick patient to a PHYSIOLOGICAL (healthy) CAT I. So, the CAT II or CAT III must be returned to CAT I status, and then the CAT I must be cleard of distortion. Remember, a healthy person is in

PHYSIOLOGICAL CAT I status and should be kept that way.

Understanding SOT analysis will tell the practitioner what is causing what. The practitioner will be able to unravel the many seemingly mysterious ramifications of CSF Stenosis, SI strain, sprain and separation, as well as the many variations of vertebral joint and disc dysfunctions.

SOT procedures will offer a very effective method of correcting these faults and restoring normal function. As a student or doctor of SOT, you may choose to absorb the entire package or those parts that help to improve your skill as a Chiropractor. You must be the judge of that.

THE CERVICAL STAIRSTEP TECHNIQUE

The **CERVICAL STAIRSTEP TECHNIQUE** is a technique that can be used for any Category. With practice, it can provide information about the cervical spine; where it is functioning normally and where it is having a problem. It is also a form of gentle adjustment where necessary.

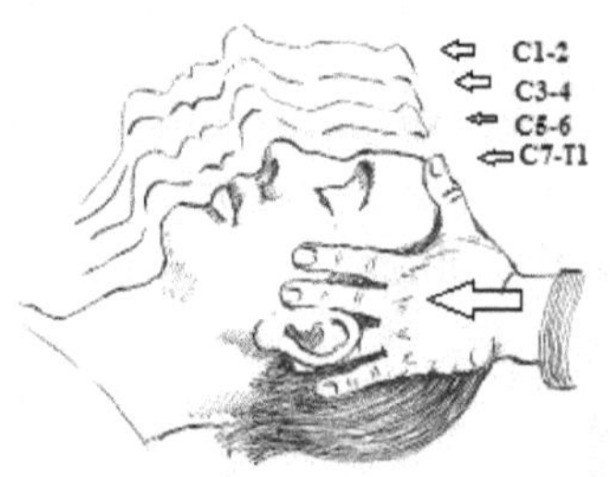

With the patient in the supine position, place both hands on the head – one on either side straddling the ears. Then apply a firm pedal (caudal) pressure. The head will gradually rise off the table while you keep the face horizontal. With practice, learn to identify four distinct fluid steps as the head rises. For example, the first step is at the level of T1/C7 (the segments tend to move in units of two). If there is resistance felt at one of the levels as the head rises from the applied pedal (caudal) pressure, then that is the level that needs to be addressed.

At the point where a stop of the upward slide is felt, hold the head at that level and move the head in a sideward's motion so the patient's chin moves in a figure eight motion or in other word, following the direction of the infinity sign (∞). Be sure to keep the head facing towards the ceiling, without rotation of the head. Once the segments are fluid in motion, continue the stair step motion to the next level, working up the cervical spine.

Many cervical misalignments will be corrected by this very simple and non-invasive low-force technique.

1

CHUNKING

In compiling these notes, the attempt is to present the material in a way that makes it easier for the field doctor who, like many, has to convert the mass of information that SOT presents into a tangible alternative to one's own approach to Chiropractic.

The sheer volume of information contained in the courses and notes is enough to overwhelm the busy practitioner, discouraging them from converting to the SOT approach. One may either make-do with a simplified version or return to the COMFORT ZONE of familiar techniques.

The rewards for the DC who perseveres with mastering SOT are tremendous. SOT offers the practitioner a diversified and logical approach to Chiropractic. It does not claim to be a panacea, nor does it do-away-with the spinal adjustment; indeed it is a very good rationale for knowing when and where to adjust and when to use other methods. The **BLOCKS** are an important part of SOT, but do not replace the hands.

In studying SOT from the notes alone, it may be found that the best method of learning the technique was through **CHUNKING**. To explain, the human brain can only retain for immediate memory a limited number of pieces of information. In order to be able to expand our knowledge, it is helpful to group pieces of information into 'chunks' and then expand upon them.

As an example, remember when you were learning to drive a car. At first the many aspects of driving a car may have seemed overwhelming: press the clutch, find first gear (is it up or down or to one side?), release the hand brake, ease up on the clutch whilst pressing down on the accelerator, glance in the rear view mirror.... the list seemed endless; an impossible mental juggling act. With practice, all that information becomes a single CHUNK called driving a car. Now, while driving a car you might engage in a conversation, notice the scenery, adjust the air conditioner or radio setting.

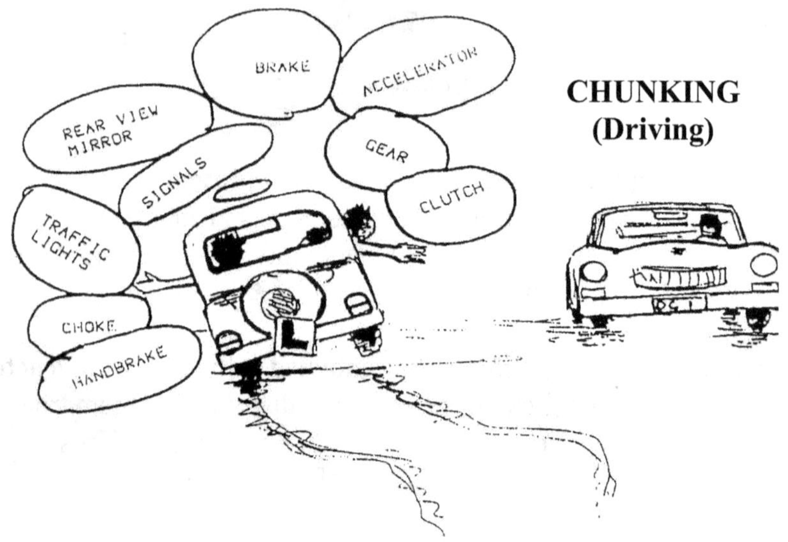

This book attempts to CHUNK the SOT system, starting with a small manageable chunk and then building onto it.

The HANDS-ON approach to learning is a must for Chiropractors and nowhere more so than with SOT. The book starts by introducing a chunk or an addition to the chunk, explains how to do it so that the practitioner can put it into practice. The explanation and rationale accompanies each chunk.

The student or doctor (of SOT) should exercise patience and truly 'chunk' each step before moving-on. The steps required to determine a Category should be automatic with no short cuts and NO STEPS LEFT OUT.

The driver cannot miss any of the steps when driving a car; every step is necessary. So it is with practicing SOT.

2

ANALYSIS

I'm assuming the people studying this work are either gratuate DC's or are Chiropractic students. If not, then I suggest putting this book back on the shelf to let it collect dust until truly in a position to put it to work on patients.

The first and very important steps to deciding which CATEGORY a new patient exhibits are within the analysis of the patient. Without apology, this chapter teaches what to do without having yet given an explanation of *why* or even *what to look for.* Learn this routine, do each and every step, and record your findings. Learn *why* later. It's like learning to drive a car: you don't need to know what is under the bonnet to start driving.

Take a careful case history and perform a normal physical examination of your patient before trying to establish a Category. A routine case history includes specific questions and answers providing clues to guide the practitioner towards finding a Category. With experience using SOT, identifying a Category becomes second nature. This will all become clear as we go along.

VISUAL EXAMINATION (PATIENT FACING DOCTOR)

The first examination is started with the patient standing facing the doctor. This is where you start to develop your observation.

Look for the following points:

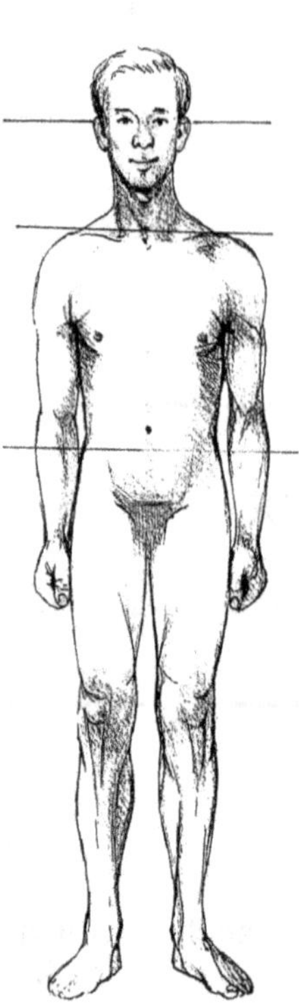

- Note the positioning of the head, and determine if one ear is high and/or more prominent than the other.
- Note the expression on the patient's face, perhaps displaying the level of pain or distress the patient is experiencing.
- Examine the shape of the head and face. Note if one eye is higher than the other, if the chin is neutral or pointing to one side, if the nose is neutral or pointing to one side.
- Note the positioning of the shoulders. Is one shoulder higher than the other? Notice if a high shoulder is high on the same side as the high ear, or if they are opposite.
- Examine the Chest and torso. Note if they are symmetrical. Does the umbilicus twist to one side? Check to see and note if the umbilicus twists to the same side as the nose.
- Examine the position of the knees, knock-kneed (genu valgus) or bowed (genu varus).

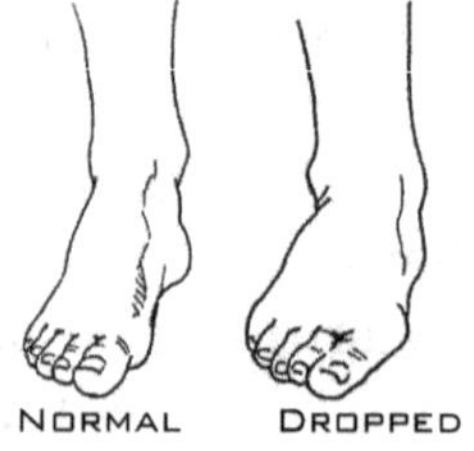

- Examine the position of the feet to note if they are angled equally. Look at the shape of the arch: is there a dropped arch? Is it unilateral or bilateral?

THE PLUMLINE EXAMINATION

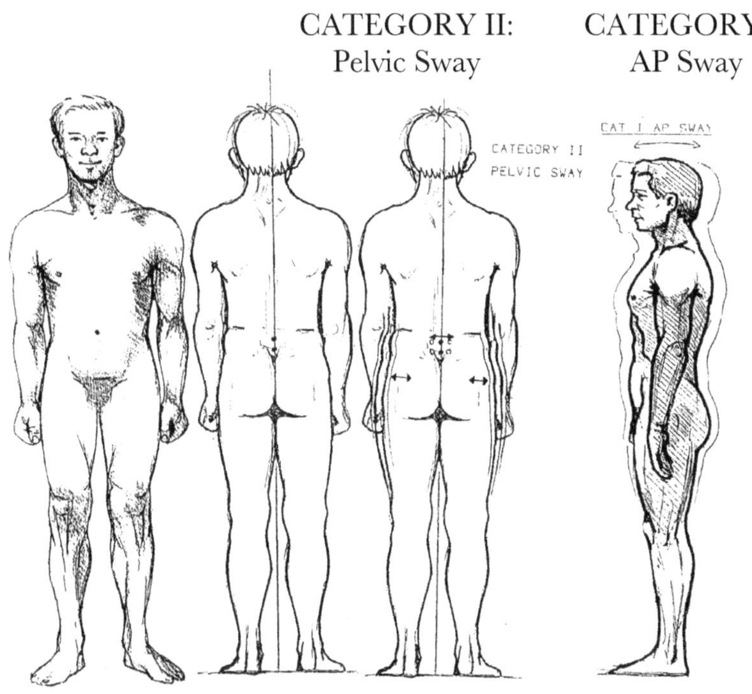

Stand the patient in front of a plumbline or at the back of a chair, so to have a fixed vertical reference to compare with their posture. Ask the patient to "stand relaxed looking straight ahead." Look for a **HIGH OCCIPUT**, **HIGH SHOULDER**, and **HIGH PELVIS**.

Now ask the patient to close their eyes, and observe what happens. Observe for any motion of the body. Be aware of how the patient moves. Is the patient relatively mobile, stiff, or obviously apprehensive?

The dots on the Sacral spinous will help determine the **LATERAL SWAY**.

Does he/she ROCK FORWARDS AND BACKWARDS (AP SWAY)? Step over to one side of the patient to further check for ANTERIOR-POSTERIOR (AP) SWAY. Do the HIPS SWAY or MOVE OFF CENTER?

Make a note of an Antalgic Lean or Loss of Lumbar Curvature. RECORD EVERYTHING YOU SAW.

MASTOID, MID CERVICALS AND 1st RIB HEADS

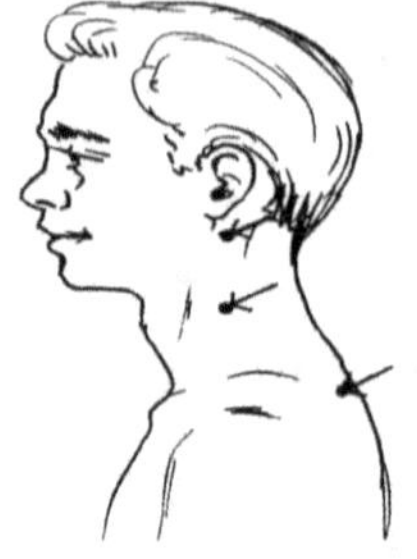

**Mastoid,
Mid-Cervicals
& Head**

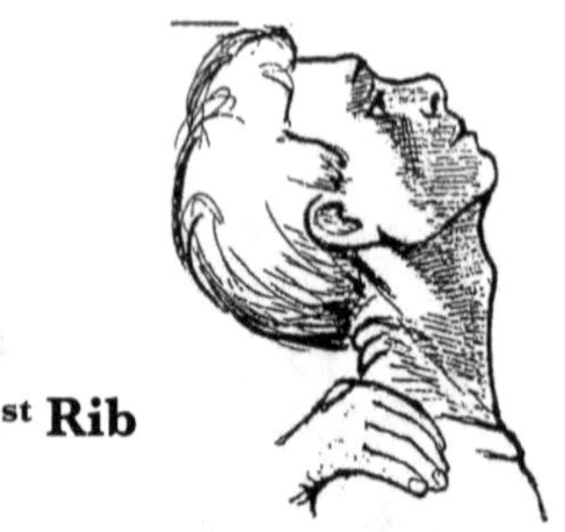

1st Rib

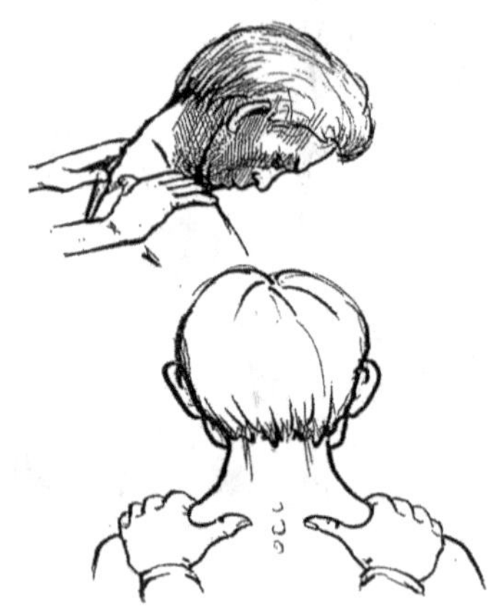

With the patient standing, reach up and palpate the tips of the **MASTOIDS**, feel for any small nodule; they may be painful.

Palpate the Transverses of the **4th CERVICAL**; look for tenderness. The references to mid cervicals and C4 are not part of the original work by Dr. De Jarnette; however, some practitioners, including the author, have noticed a correlation. I have included them for **reference only**.

Bring palpating hands down to rest across the shoulders, thumbs now over the **1ST RIB HEADS**. Feel for prominence or tenderness. Ask the patient to bend the head forward with neck flexion and then backwards with neck extension. Feel for any movement of the rib heads, either one side or both.

This is also a good position to feel for and look for tension and muscle imbalance in the trapezius muscles.

RECORD EVERYTHING YOU SAW AND FELT.

THE MIND LANGUAGE TEST

The patient is still in the standing position with their back to the doctor, feet apart, eyes looking straight ahead. Make sure the jaw is relaxed and not tightly clenched. Ask the patient to raise the right arm out to the side (shoulder abduction), with the arm level to the floor and fist clenched.

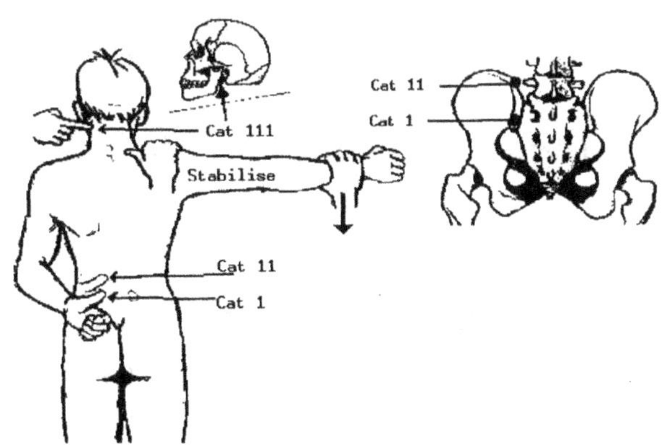

The doctor LEFT HAND is placed on the patient's RIGHT SHOULDER (to stabalize the test) and the other hand over the patient's RIGHT WRIST (to apply the pressure to perform the test). The doctor's thumb should not fully grasp the wrist but merely support the underside of it.

Explain to the patient: "When I say **'HOLD'** I will push down on the wrist and I want you to resist my pressure so that your arm does not drop." Try the test with the patient. If the patient does not fully understand, patiently explain the directions again until the patient exhibits a strong resistance to the pressure applied at the wrist.

Remember this is a **TEST,** not a contest.

Now, with the LEFT HAND grasp the thumb of the patient's LEFT HAND (opposite the testing arm) and guide it back to touch and press on their LEFT PSIS. With the patient maintaining a firm **pressure on the PSIS**, return your LEFT HAND to the patient's RIGHT SHOULDER and your RIGHT HAND to the patient's RIGHT WRIST, and again command **'HOLD'** to test the response.

Guide the patient's LEFT THUMB up to the **CREST OF THE ILIUM** just lateral to the mamillary process of L5. Again command **'HOLD'** to test the response.

Bring the patient's hand up to the left side of his face and place their pointed INDEX FINGER as close to or on the **STYLOID PROCESS.** With the patient maintaining a reasonable pressure on the **STYLOID PROCESS** (this is a sensitive area, so don't press too hard), again command **'HOLD'** to test the response.

SUPINE & PRONE EXAMINATION

Whether the doctor chooses to examine the patient Supine or Prone first is their own choice and will depend on the findings from the standing tests, particularly the MIND LANGUAGE TEST. The supine & prone tests are used in addition to any other orthopedic tests routinely performed.

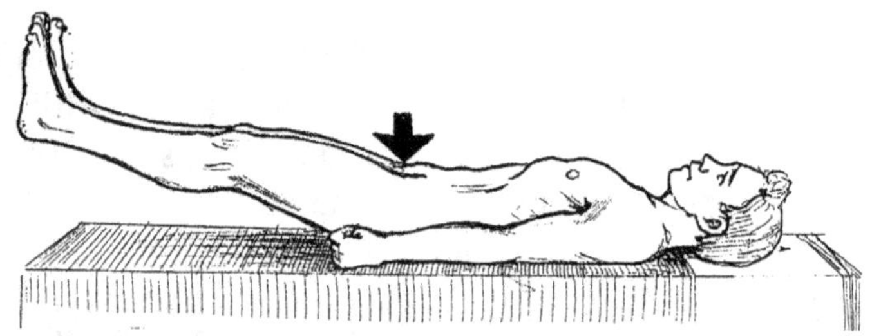

SUPINE - STRAIGHT LEG RAISES

While the patient is lying SUPINE, ask them to raise both legs straight up off the table without using their hands, (heels raised approximately 18 inches off of the table is sufficient). Watch what happens. Look at the patient's face: is there any sign of strain or distress? The patient may not be able to raise their legs at all or may do so with ease.

The patient lowers the legs. Place one hand firmly on the patient's PUBIS and ask him to raise the legs again.

Was it more difficult with pubic support or without?

RECORD EVERYTHING YOU FOUND.

Go to the head of the table and place both hands on the patient's head, just above the ears. Without any pressure being exerted ask the patient to raise both legs exactly the same amount as the Straight Leg Raise test. Take note of the effort required and any discomfort.

After the patient has lowered the legs, exert a **PEDAL (caudal) PRESSURE** causing **CERVICAL COMPACTION** and ask the patient to raise the legs once more. Which test was more difficult for the patient to do?

RECORD WHAT HAPPENED.

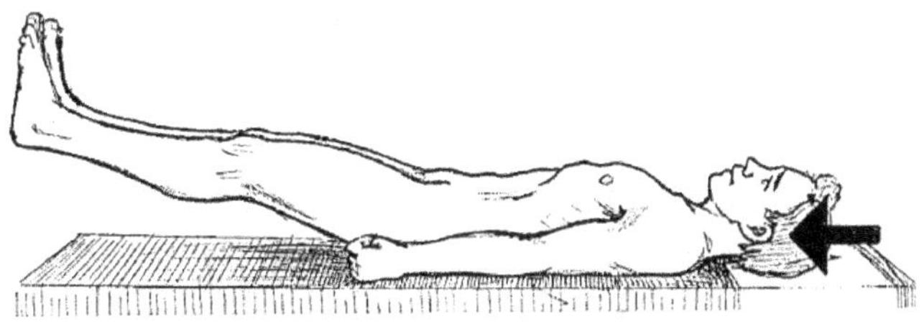

I am assuming that you will incorporate your routine ORTHOPEDIC and NEUROLOGICAL TESTS where appropriate.

AS A DOCTOR OF CHIROPRACTIC, YOU MUST BE ABLE TO ASCERTAIN THE FULL HEALTH PICTURE OF THE PATIENT, AND BE ABLE TO DETECT ANY PROBLEM THAT REQUIRES A CHIROPRACTIC APPROACH, AS WELL AS ANY PROBLEM THAT MAY BE MORE APPROPRIATELY CARED FOR BY ANOTHER HEALTH PROFESSIONAL.

SUPINE – THE ARM FOSA TEST

This test is specifically for the CAT II but it is a good habit to involve it in the routine test, often you will detect a CAT II, which may not have presented using solely the Mind Language Test.

INGUINAL LIGAMENT:

The UPPER HALF of the INGUINAL LIGAMENT relates to the UPPER FOSSA and the LOWER HALF relates to the LOWER FOSSA.

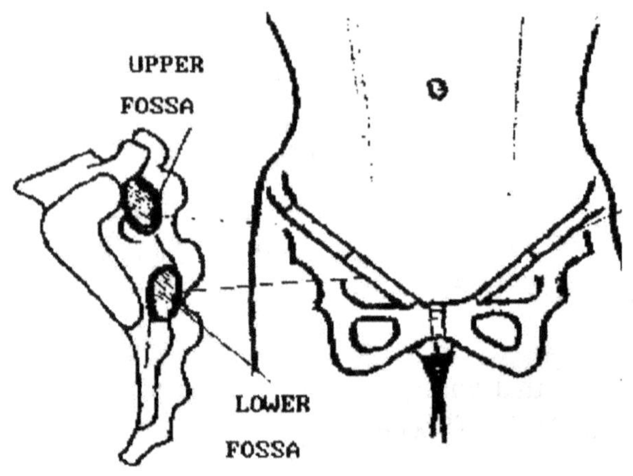

Having completed the **CERVICAL COMPACTION TEST**, move to the patient's LEFT SIDE. Stand level with the patient's LEFT HIP, angling your stance cephalad to face the patient's RIGHT SHOULDER. Raise the patient's LEFT ARM vertically in shoulder flexion; and ask the patient to make a fist and **'HOLD'** the arm in that position. Your RIGHT HAND grasps the patient's WRIST with the fingers above and the thumb below. The thumb should not grasp the wrist tightly; it should be there only to keep the fingers in place.

Explain to the patient: "I am going to press your arm down towards your feet and I want you to resist my pressure." In the application of pressure, press with a flat hand using the fingers only.

Say: "When I say **'HOLD'** (or **LOCK**) resist my pressure." Be sure that the patient understands. If necessary, repeat the instructions until the patient understands.

With the first finger of your LEFT HAND, palpate the Anterior Spine of the **LEFT ILIUM**. Bring all four fingers down to contact the **INGUINAL (Poupart's) LIGAMENT**. To do this, slide the first finger just medial to the **ASIS** and then bring the other fingers so that the tips are pressed evenly along the ligament.

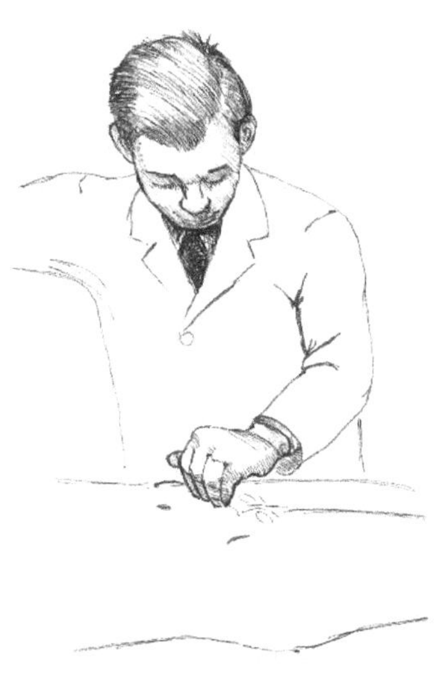

Having found the right place, which should be along the lateral half of the Inguinal Ligament, ease the pressure so that the fingers are merely resting on the surface of the skin.

Say: **'HOLD', and simultaneously maintain contact on the INGUINAL LIGAMENT while pressing the test ARM in a PEDAL (caudal) ARC** (just far enough to feel the patient's response). It is not a contest of strength; be able to feel the difference between a strong and a weak response compared with the first test performed before contacting the Inguinal Ligament.

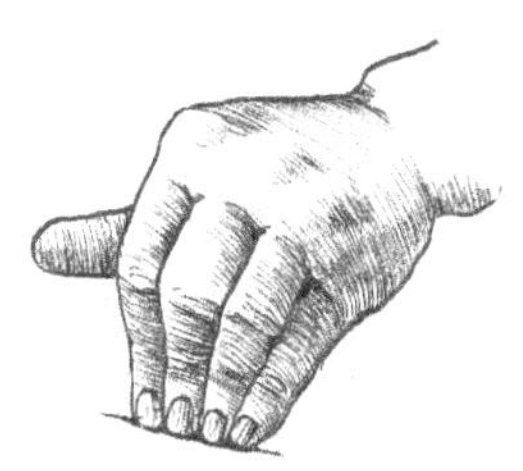

Slide the contact hand caudally down the INGUINAL (Poupart's) LIGAMENT until the little finger touches the **PUBIS** at the **distal end of the INGUINAL LIGAMENT**. Remove your contact hand and perform a preliminary test. Then, repeat the **TEST with contact.** Say: **'HOLD', and simultaneously maintain contact on the distal portion of the INGUINAL LIGAMENT while pressing the test ARM in a PEDAL (caudal) ARC.**

Compare responses. If the first test (without making contact) was weak, this creates a problem (and will deal with that a little later). The first test is the **NORM** for the particular side tested that the two Inguinal Ligament tests are compared to.

Walk CLOCK-WISE around the table. Take up a similar position on the LEFT side of the patient and go through the same routine. (Walk *ANTI-CLOCK-WISE in the Southern hemisphere.)

UMS/LLL Remember this formula. An **Upper** fossa weakness corresponds with **Medial** leg pain and the **Short** leg (UMS). A **Lower** fossa weakness corresponds with **Lateral** leg knee pain and the **Long** leg (LLL). If this formula is not present, recheck the fossa and leg lengths; and if still not correct, then check for other problems, such as Psoas, Diaphragm or Upper Cervicals.

PRONE EXAMINATION

Beyond a normal Chiropractic examination and palpation, the items to look for in the **PRONE** position include:

Heal Tension	**Covered under CAT I**
Short Leg	**CAT I & III, differentiate from Anatomical SL, Atlas/Axis etc.**
Muscle Wasting	**CAT III**
Quadratus Lumborum Tension	**CAT I: CRESTS**
Gluteals	**CAT I: DOLLARS**

THE SET OF TESTS PERFORMED IN THE STANDING, SUPINE AND PRONE POSITIONS ARE IN NO WAY THE ENTIRE PACKAGE. HAVING COME THIS FAR IN THE EXAMINATION, THE DOCTOR SHOULD HAVE SOME IDEA OF THE NATURE OF THE PATIENT'S PROBLEM AND ENOUGH KNOWLEDGE TO IDENTIFY THE CATEGORY. MORE TESTS WILL BE REQUIRED TO EXPLORE THE INDIVIDUAL CATEGORY.

REVIEW

TEST	FINDINGS
Standing, Plumbline Visualization	
Mastoid, Mid-Cervical, 1st Rib Head	
Mind Language	
Leg Raise, Pubic Contact	
Cervical Compaction Test	
Fossa Test	

At this point, be content to incorporate these tests into a normal routine examination.

······· DO NOT GO ON UNTIL YOU HAVE 'CHUNKED' ·······

3

INTERPRETING THE TESTS

This chapter delves into quite a bit of detail about the interpretation of the tests performed. Use this section as reference material. As you become used to doing the tests you will gradually learn what each means. Continue doing the tests even if uncertain of their relevance.

By the time the patient is ready for examination standing in front of the doctor, several observations have already been made. The doctor has been talking to the patient during the consultation and disclosed their complaint(s); however, more visually, the doctor has also witnessed the patient walking in to the room, sitting down – perhaps reluctantly. Also observed were the patient's facial expressions and their general bearing during the consultation. To the observant doctor all these things have started to paint a picture.

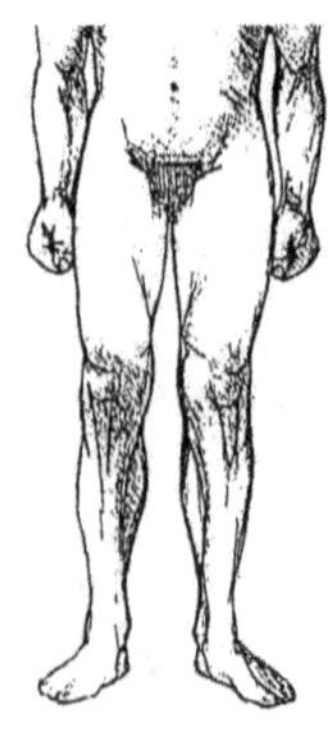

PATIENT STANDING

HIPS

Are the HIPS even, high on one side, or displaced to one side? An Antalgic Lean would lead the doctor to think of a disc problem and CAT III.

FEET & KNEES

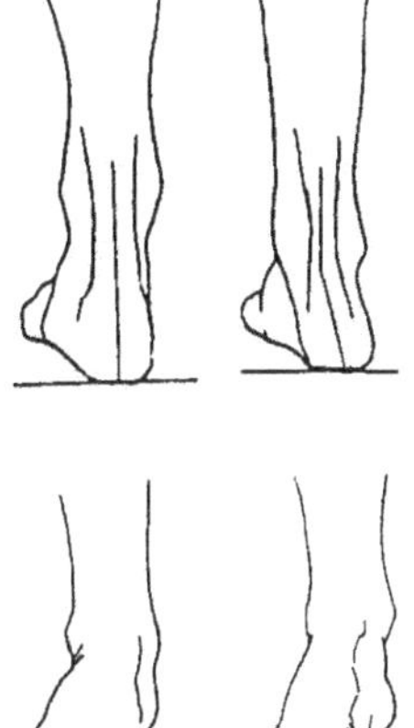

With the patient facing the doctor, glance down at the FEET and KNEES. Look at the angle of the feet, (ideally 45°). Are they equally angled? Do the arches look high, normal or dropped? The angle of the feet can be indicative of pelvic distortion. Arch drop can cause or be caused by Sacral weakness. The knee will usually accompany the weak arch sagging medially.

SHOULDERS

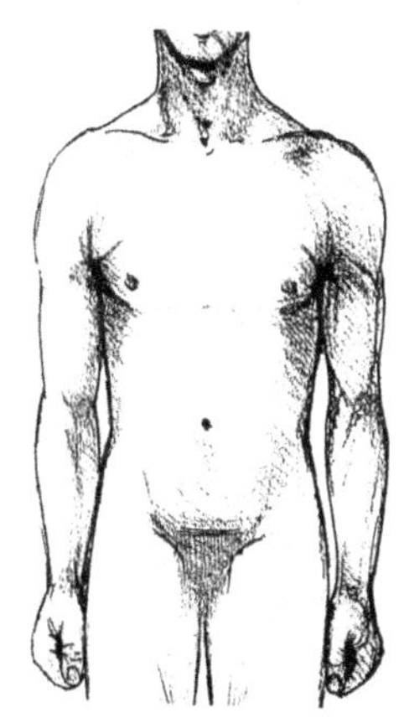

Are the SHOULDERS level? If one is high, is it on the same side as the high hip, or opposite side?

A high ear on the same side as a high shoulder indicates a possible **Condyle Subluxation.**

If the patient is showing signs of CAT II, but has the high ear/high shoulder, then test for the **Condyle Subluxation** and clear it before proceeding with CAT II Blocking. After clearing the Condyle Subluxation, the CAT II tests may have also cleared.

UMBILICUS

Look at the UMBILICUS. Is it central, or does it seem to be twisted to one side? If displaced, the umbilicus usually swings towards the side of the SHORT LEG.

FACE

Look at the symmetry of the FACE. If you keep looking at the bone structure of your patients' faces you will soon notice asymmetrical faces, eyes uneven, nose twisted and jaw swung to one side. If displaced, the NOSE AND JAW will usually swing towards the side of the SHORT LEG.

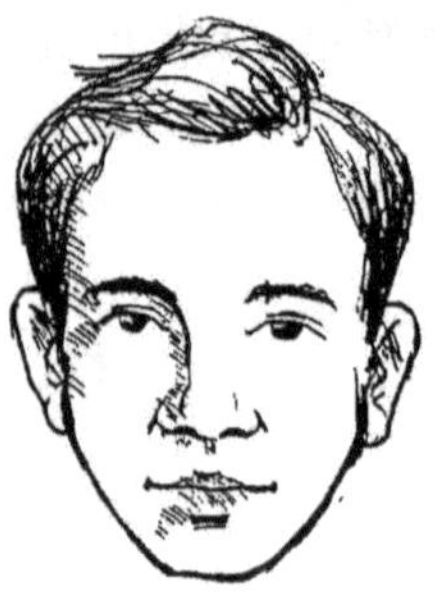

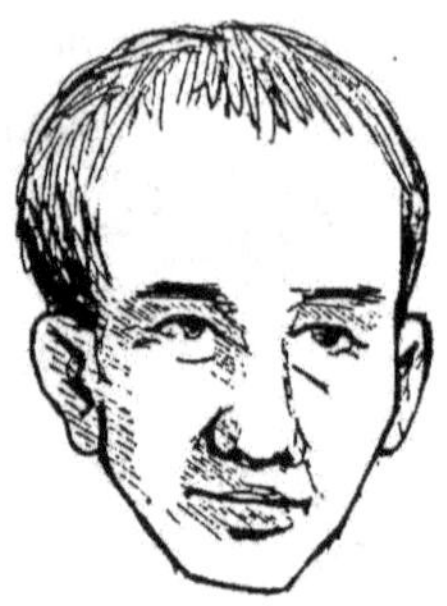

Is one ear more prominent than the other? All of these are points to recognize and will become of use when applying Cranial Adjusting.

VISUALIZING WITH THE PLUMBLINE

Ideally there should be two plumblines between the doctor and the patient. This helps to ensure that any swaying or movement can be differentiated between that of the patient and that of the doctor. The patient's feet should be slightly apart, with the heels level. A specially designed footboard can be used.

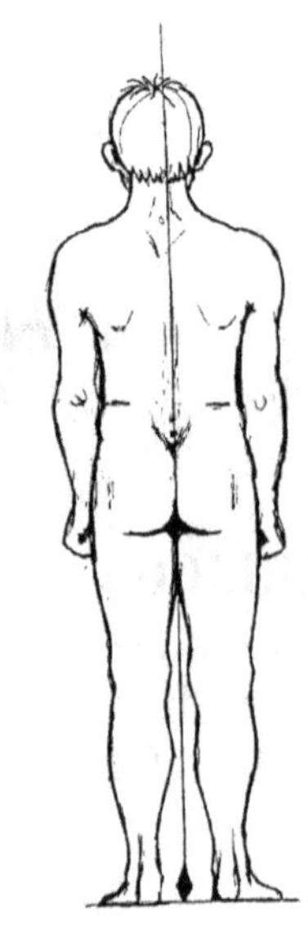

The full spine and the pelvis should be visible for inspection. It helps to use a skin pencil to mark at least two points down the Sacral spinouses. With the patient standing, weight equally distributed, position the patient so that the gap between the feet is bisected by the plumbline and the Sacral Crest is in line.

Bring the pelvis central if necessary; then allow the patient to find his own level again. **WATCH WHAT HAPPENS.**

Does the pelvis appear rigid? (CAT I) Does the patient sway from side to side or just swing to one side? (CAT II).

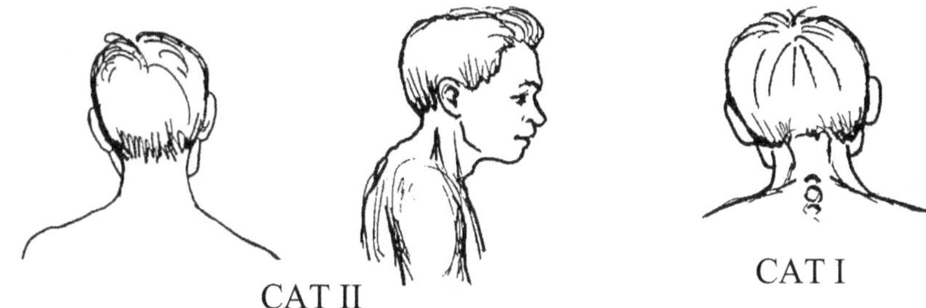

CAT II CAT I

Look at the way the patient holds the head. The CAT I tends to carry his head as if it were too heavy; usually the Occiput is low on one side. The Atlas is always involved in the CAT I complex. The Occiput is often low on one side with the chin pointing towards the high side in a CAT II.

A-P SWAY

If the patient starts to sway forward and backward when asked to close the eyes, this is a further indication of a CAT I complex. As the locking of the pelvic motion has impaired the normal res-piratory mechanism, the body responds by rocking the spine to try to maintain the CSF pump mechanism.

LUMBAR POSTURE

The standing posture of the patient was revealed during the examination. Take specific note whether there is any ANTALGIC LEAN or LOSS OF or INCREASE IN NORMAL LUMBAR LORDOSIS.

CAT I: If the patient stands erect with some degree of scoliosis and shoulder drop, PLUS a HEAVY LOOKING HEAD, then a CAT I is suspected.

CAT II: An unstable pelvis, either floating from side to side or just to one side and a LOSS OF LUMBAR LORDOSIS, we can consider the CAT II. There is often that look of distress especially when walking or rising from a chair.

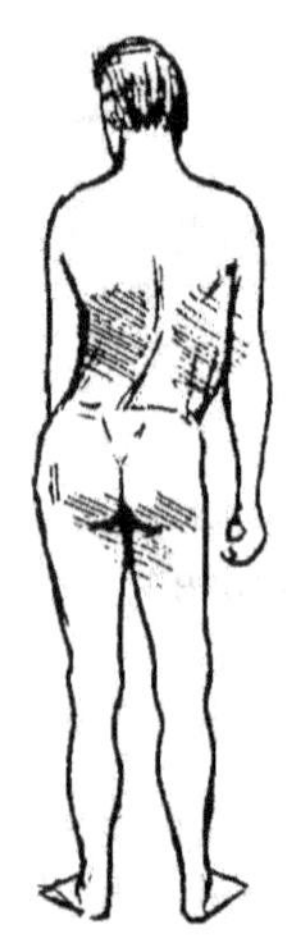

CAT III: The SCIATICA patient often exhibits a dramatic ANTALGIC LEAN as the body tries to minimize the irritation to the nerve or cord. Make a careful note whether the lean is towards or away from the side of sciatica. This is an important consideration when it comes to adjusting, and is discussed in the management of a CAT III case.

MASTOID, 4TH CERVICAL & 1ST RIB HEAD

MASTOID

Slide the first finger of each hand down the MASTOIDS to the very tip and feel for a small nodule, often a bit sore. Ask the patient which side is more painful; it will probably coincide with the side with a palpable nodule. This is a **CAT II indicator**.

MASSETER MUSCLES

Reach around to the patient's cheeks and press the anterior margins of the MASSETER MUSCLES, just above the lower teeth, and ask the patient to open his mouth.

One side may be quite tender, this is another **CAT II indicator**, but it also **indicates a TMJ problem** (often part of a CAT II complex). This was not part of the original CHUNK but comes into play later.

MID CERVICAL

Pass the fingers down the CERVICAL SPINE and palpate for a tight painful area just anterior to the 4th Cervical vertebra, ask the patient which side is more painful, you will usually be able to tell him, but ask anyway. This is another **CAT II indicator**.

1st RIB HEAD

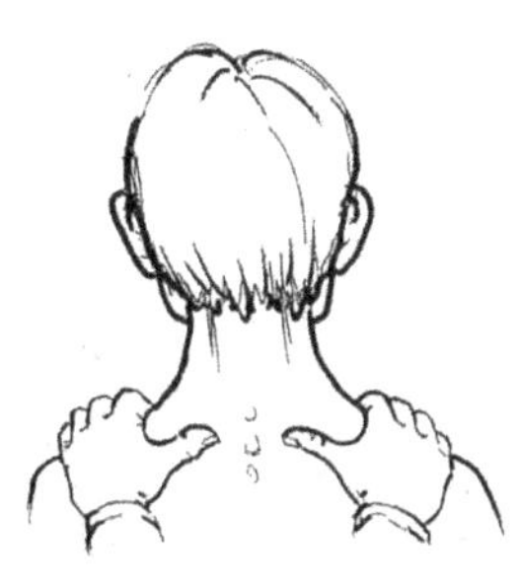

Place both hands lightly on the shoulders, thumbs pointing inwards. The tips of the thumbs should be just over the 1st RIB HEADS. Palpate for a prominent rib head; it may be painful. Ask the patient to bend their head forward in hyper-flexion. Now ask the patient to bring the head all the way back into Hyperextension. Feel for motion of the 1st RIB HEADS.

Normally, there would NOT be any motion. However, in the case of a **CAT I** there will be motion on **BOTH RIBS**. In the case of a **CAT II, ONE RIB HEAD will be prominent, painful and mobile.**

MUSCLE TESTING

Muscle testing is now used in various health fields and has become a useful tool for Chiropractors and Kinesiologists alike. At first glance it appears somewhat esoteric and so worthy of skepticism. However, with acceptance of the information that this type of testing can provide, a whole new avenue of examination opens up. Remember, no single test should be taken as a definitive diagnosis. The tests used in SOT are part of the solution to a puzzle and only when all the pieces (or at least a good many of them) fit into place can the picture be seen.

Learn to include muscle testing into your routine. Patients will accept it and will be interested by the findings. Patients also learn to recognize that as their condition improves so do the tests.

Make sure that the test arm is strong before starting a test. Occasionally, the patient may have a shoulder problem or a weak muscle, which can make the test difficult. In this case, use the opposite side to perform the test. The test is just as valid with the left arm as it is with the right arm.

There are times when the patient is unable to stand for the test, in which case the patient may be tested lying prone. When there is obvious difficulty with patient cooperation or when the patient is very old and frail, then a **SURROGATE TESTER** may be used (See Surrogate Testing Section).

MIND LANGUAGE TEST

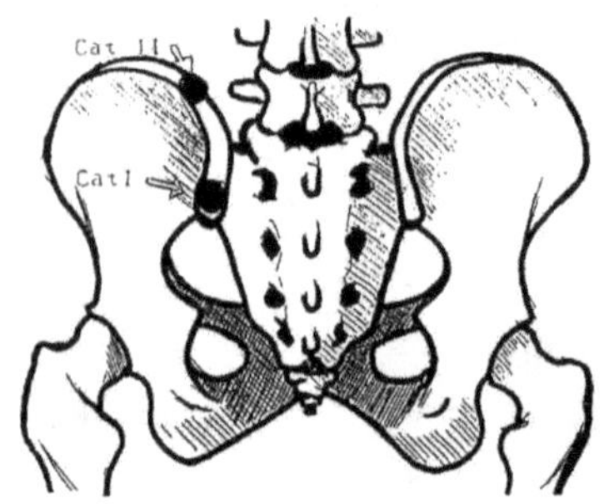

If the testing arm goes weak when the first contact point is pressed at the **PSIS**, this indicates a **CAT I**.

If weak on the second point at the **Crest of the Ilium** close to the spinous of the 5th Lumbar, then a **CAT II** is suspected.

Mind Language CAT I & II

CAT III

Weakness of the **Styloid Process** contact would indicate a **CAT III**. You can identify the particular vertebra by putting the contact onto the transverse or mamillary process of each lumbar segment.

4TH & 5TH LUMBAR

While in the Mind Language position, ask the patient to slightly bend the right knee and test the arm for strength and then do the same with the left leg.

A weakness of the arm during knee flexion would indicate a 4th or 5th Lumbar posterior junction involvement, but more on this later.

SUPINE TESTS

LEGS RAISING WITHOUT/WITH PUBIS SUPPORT

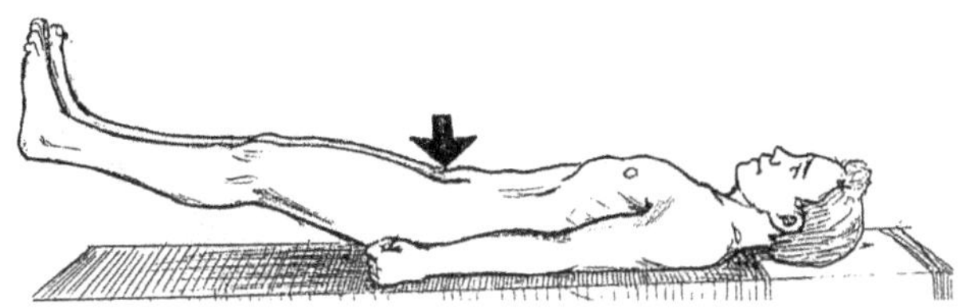

Make sure the patient does not use the hands to press down against the table. If he finds it EASIER to raise the legs **WHEN THE PUBIS IS PRESSED** this is a **CAT II indicator**. By pressing on the pubis you are giving the pelvis more stability. Without the pubis support the strain of lifting the legs is localized in the pelvis; and in the presence of a weakened Sacroiliac, the strain is greater.

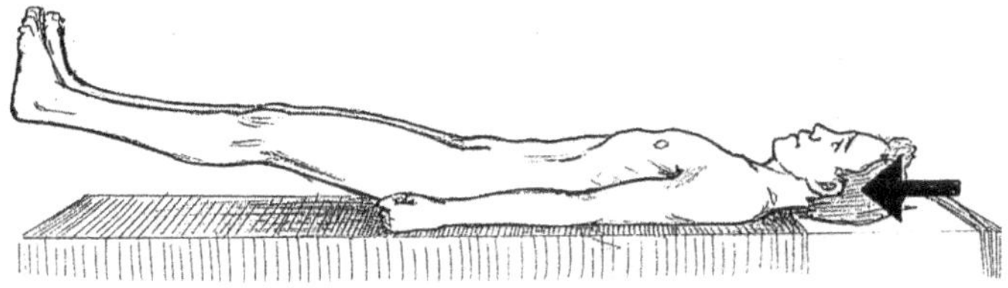

If there is difficulty in raising the legs but the Pubic pressure did not make a difference, then the **CERVICAL COMPACTION TEST** may show a **Cervical involvement**.

Once the neck has been stabilized by the doctor's pressure the body can then exert sufficient strength to raise the legs.

When there is difficulty raising the legs with light contact at the head without any pressure and **made easier** with the addition of **CERVICAL COMPACTION** pressure to the head, this is a **CERVICAL INDICATOR**. Once the neck has been stabilized by the doctor's pressure the body can then exert sufficient strength to raise the legs.

If the patient can raise the legs without CERVICAL pressure, but finds it more **difficult with CERVICAL COMPACTION** then it is a **CAT II indicator.**

ADDITIONAL TESTS IN THE SUPINE POSITION

There are two tests that you can do to look for a weak **PSOAS**.

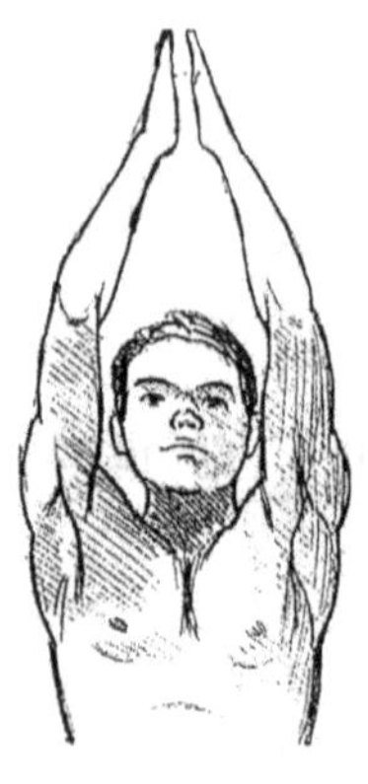

1. De Jarnette Psoas Test: Ask the patient to raise both arms above the head and turn the hands so that the fingers are parallel and the palms are facing each other. Grasp both wrists and pull slightly to make sure that the body is straight. **Look to see whether one arm is longer than the other.**

There is some difference of opinion as to whether to regard the SHORT ARM side as being a PSOAS IN CONTRACTION or the LONG ARM side as being a WEAK PSOAS. I usually identify the WEAK PSOAS with use of the AK testing. The Psoas in spasm is a real variation, but a muscle in spasm is in fact a weak muscle, so keep an open mind and make a decision case by case.

2. AK Psoas Muscle Test: To do this test, stand on the side of the leg being tested and raise the leg straight to about 45° from the floor and then ABDUCT the leg about 45° from the midline. With one hand holding the leg, place the other hand on the OPPOSITE ANTERIOR CREST OF THE ILIUM. Explain to the patient that you are going to press the leg DOWN AND OUT and you want him to resist UP AND MEDIAL. Compare the two sides.

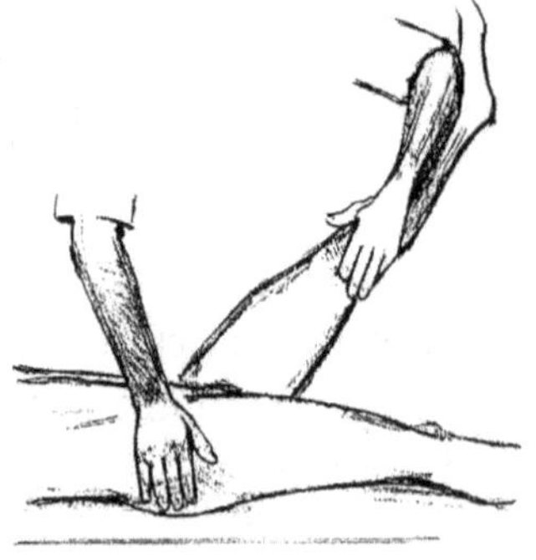

9TH THORACIC

This is an additional test not yet discussed. It is mentioned in this discussion so as to offer a context for its later use.

With the patient still in the supine position, ask him to raise one leg six to eight inches off of the table and ask him to resist downward pressure to the leg. Then test the other leg. Look to find a weak side.

Confirm by asking the patient to bend one knee with the foot on the table, and perform the test on the leg OPPOSITE of the bent knee. A weakness will be more apparent. A **weakness** here means a possible **9T DURAL TORQUE** involvement.

ARM FOSSA TEST

The ARM FOSSA TEST is not a simple muscle test. There is a complex neurological involvement requiring perception of the COMMAND 'HOLD' (perceived by the brain) simultaneously with the proprioceptive messages of the CHALLENGE at the INGUINAL LIGAMENT and the ARM FEELING THE PRESSURE (perceived by the cerebellum). The Brain literally tells the arm not to resist when the Challenge to an Inguinal ligament causes an alarm signal to the proprioceptors in the corresponding Sacroiliac fossa.

When one or more of the four points of Challenge along the Inguinal (Poupart's) Ligaments causes a weakness in the testing arm, this is a strong indicator for a **CAT II.**

CONDYLES

If there is a HIGH EAR on the same side as the HIGH SHOULDER, then it would be expedient at this point to test for a CONDYLE SUBLUXATION.

Go to the head of the patient; ask him to raise the RIGHT arm to the vertical and make a fist. Explain: "I am going to pull your arm *headward* and I want you to resist." Once there is a good resistance, go to the LEFT MASTOID just behind the ear and press caudally with the thumb – so as to force the skull (condyle) down onto the Atlas; with this pressure, test the RIGHT arm. Then, slide the finger below the LEFT MASTOID and pull it upward – so as to pull the LEFT CONDYLE away from the Atlas; with this pressure, test the RIGHT arm. Repeat this on the RIGHT CONDYLE whilst testing the LEFT ARM.

A weak arm will indicate a condyle involvement according to the challenge. If the pressure down towards the Atlas causes a weakness, then the CONDYLE is subluxated low on that side. The line of force for the corrective adjustment must be in the opposite direction of the pressure causing the weakness. Once the CONDYLE SUBLUXATION is removed, recheck the CAT II indicators; often they have been cleared out as well.

REVIEW OF THE CATEGORIES

TEST	CAT I	CAT II	CAT III
PATIENT STANDING			
A-P Sway	✓		
Lateral Pelvic Sway (Sideways)		✓	
Antalgic Lean With Sciatica			✓
Mastoid, C4 Pain		✓	
Unilateral Rib-Head Pain & Motion		✓	
Bilateral Rib-Head Pain & Motion	✓		
Mind Language			
PSIS	✓		
CREST		✓	
STYLOID			✓
PATIENT SUPINE			
Leg Raise WEAK (Pubic Support)		✓	
Cervical Compression			
WEAK with Head Pressure		✓	
STRONG With Head Pressure			**Cervical**
Arm Fossa - One Or More Weak		✓	
Psoas Weak	✓	✓	✓

THERE ARE ADDITIONAL TESTS TO ADD IN THE PROGRESSION OF TREATMENT, BUT MASTER THESE TESTS FIRST AND BECOME USED TO USING THEM AS PART OF NORMAL ROUTINE.

DISCUSSION

Once the patient has gone through the first lot of tests in the examination, the doctor should have a fair indication of the classification of the patient's CATEGORY and recognize the various symptoms of each. Do not be too hasty; this is not a simple decision. There are many variables and a careful case history is essential.

Start the observation of the patient the moment he walks into the room:

How does he walk?

How does he sit? Sometimes he may not want to sit.

Look at the facial expression, the pallor of the face and the tension of the shoulders. Hands can tell their own story.

Use your powers of observation to get as clear a picture as you can from the patient.

These are all clues, but do not be too quick to jump to conclusions. It is possible to arrive at a wrong diagnosis and then lose objectivity during the tests.

SOT makes the doctor think. The tests will help guide the doctor towards knowing what to do and when to do it, and just as importantly when to stop or do nothing.

As mentioned, the object of any procedure in SOT is to return the patient to the state of a normal **PHYSIOLOGICAL CAT I**. When there is a **CAT II** or **CAT III** they must be dealt with first; once the patient has responded and is stabilizing, he must be assessed by **CAT I** procedure until adverse signs are eliminated.

The following chapters discuss **CAT II** and **CAT III**. If the doctor can start to correct these two devastating problems, the correction will be doing a lot of good for a lot of people. Do not expect a simple two-plus-two - equals four type of equation, as there is a lot of overlapping; and be aware each category can show a highly varied pattern of symptomatology.

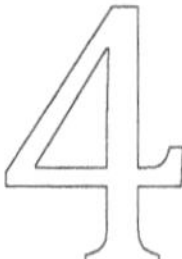

CATEGORY II

DEFINED

The CATEGORY II problem involves loss of integrity of the weight bearing interosseous part of the Sacro-iliac articulation. The problem can be a serious **SEPARATION** of one articular surface from another at the interosseous (hyaline), superior and posterior part of the articulation. It can be a **SPRAIN** causing weakness and mobility of the interosseous attachment, with increased fluid in the hyaline cartilage. Or it can be a **STRAIN** due to overloading of the weight-bearing structure. This is usually the type that has chronic and diversified symptoms.

The CAT II patient, in its many disguises, is a very common visitor to the Chiropractor's office. CAT II arrives as an **acute low back pain**, often crippling in its intensity. It comes as a **weak back** that never seems to go away. Often, the CAT II patient comes in complaining of a **neck and shoulder pain or headache,** or **nagging pain in the thoracic spine**. Because a myriad of the symptoms may present, it is good chiropractic practice to test every patient for the full range of Categories.

If any, few people reach the age of puberty without having had some type of trauma to the Sacro-iliac joint; and the cause of the various health problems plaguing them for the entirety of their lives can be detected by the oh-so-simple **Mind Language Test.**

To a large extent, the stability of the human frame depends on a stable pelvis. The muscles to the trunk, shoulders and neck originate at the pelvis. Also, the muscles to the buttocks and thighs originate at the pelvis. If the integrity of the pelvis is lost, these major muscles of support and locomotion lose their solid foundation. The abundance of proprioceptors in the Sacro-iliac Joint send distress signals that affect the proprioceptor neurons of the **Temporal Lobe** of the brain and also the **Temporal Fossa** of the temporo-mandibular articulation.

A thorough understanding of the CAT II problem can be of great assistance in the Chiropractic office. It is a very common malady and can create some of the most devastating symptoms.

Suffice it at this point to mention a most important and all too frequent fellow traveler, the **TMJ problem**, in its many varieties. A chronic CAT II will (almost without exception) be accompanied by a TMJ problem. This very important aspect of the CAT II complex is discussed later. At this point make a mental note of the **TMJ connection** and keep an eye open for signs of **TMJ problems** such as clicking, grinding or pain on chewing. As this is such a major indicator of a **CAT II,** it is essential to recognize it and later correct it and/or recommend dental cooperation.

Cat II CASE HISTORY

Your initial tests have brought you to the conclusion that the patient is suffering from a **CATEGORY II problem**. This case history is a review of what might be found in those tests.

LOW BACK

- Acute pain in the Low Back
- A feeling of severe weakness in the Low Back
- Pain may worsen when standing
- Steps are guarded and short
- Pin on turning in bed
- Difficulty getting started in the morning
- Difficulty getting up from a chair, takes a while to stand straight
- Pains into the groin and anterior or lateral thigh

OTHER SYMPTOMATOLOGY

- Neck, shoulder and arm pains/neuralgia
- Headaches
- Upper Thoracic pains
- TMJ pain, clicking or bruxism
- Knee Pain

Patients may present for a variety of seemingly unrelated reasons, yet during the examination CAT II indicators start flashing. Listen to them, as the CAT II problem can be the root cause for a multitude of ills; recognize it and correct it, and you will have done the patient a great service.

CAT II - THE STANDING PATIENT

The CAT II patient may have difficulty standing erect, walks and stands with the knees slightly bent and the shoulder and head stooped forwards, the **LUMBAR LORDOSIS** lost or diminished. One or both arches might be dropped and the knee or knees may be medially angled. There may be a toeing-in or out of one foot with or without arch drop.

MASTOID TIP

There may have been a painful nodule at the tip of one mastoid process.

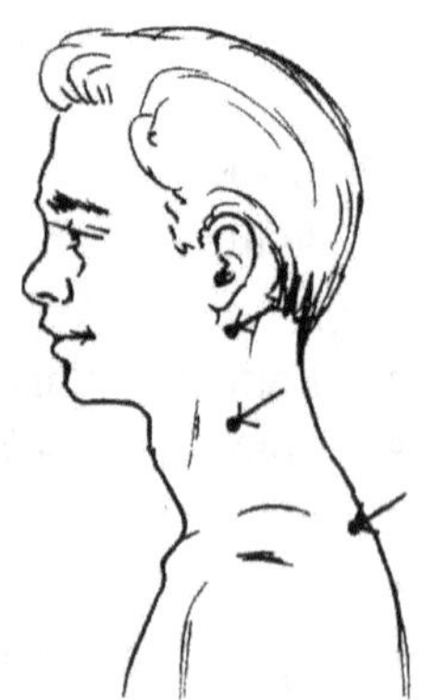

MASSETER MUSCLE

Pain may have been in the belly of one masseter muscle.

MID CERVICALS

A painful nodulation may have been found anterior to the transverse of C4.

1st RIB

One Rib Head was found to be sore, prominent & mobile.

AT THE PLUMBLINE

The pelvis does not hold steady; it either swings aimlessly or when the doctor guides the Sacrum to the center line then lets go the Sacrum swings to one side.

The Occiput is low on one side with the chin pointing to the opposite side.

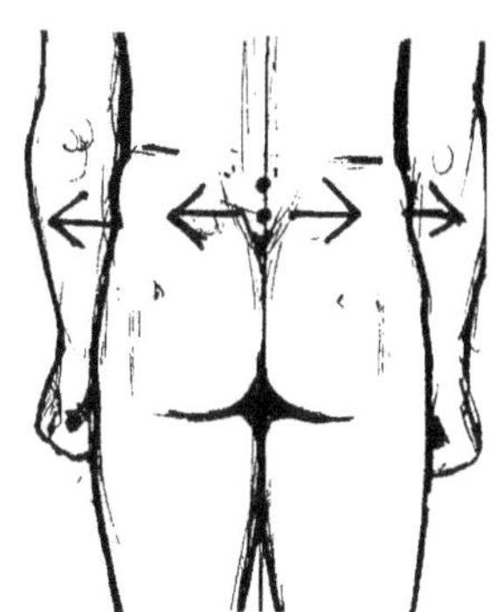

THE MIND LANGUAGE TEST

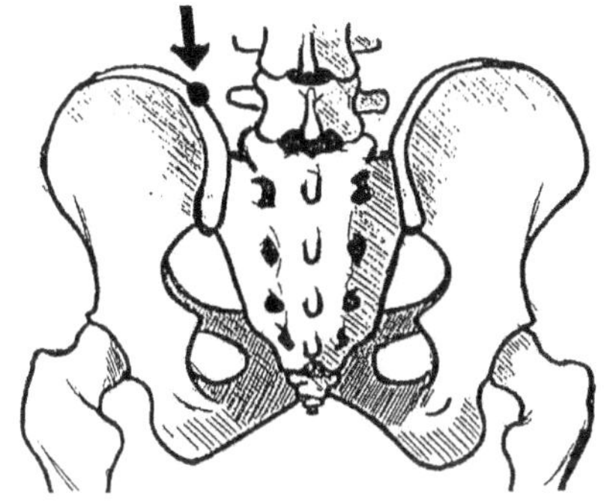

A previously strong arm goes weak when the patient contacts the **CREST OF THE ILIUM** just lateral to the Transverse of L5.

CAT II - THE SUPINE PATIENT

SUPINE LEG RAISE WITH PUBIC PRESSURE

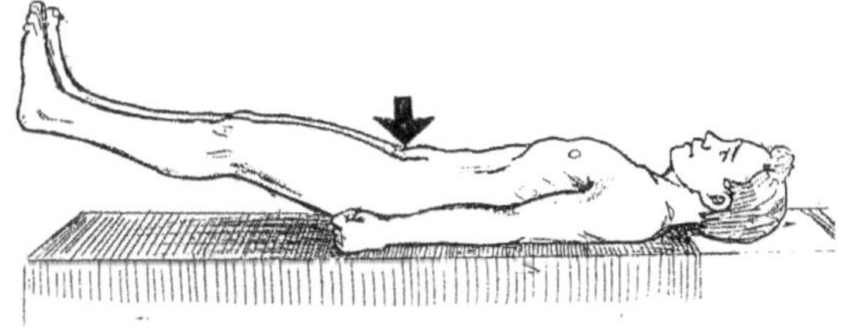

In the supine position the legs are more difficult to raise without the doctor's hand applying pressure onto the pubis. This isolates the movement at the pelvis and so the weak Sacro-iliac objects to the leg movement. Doctor's pressure gives the SI support.

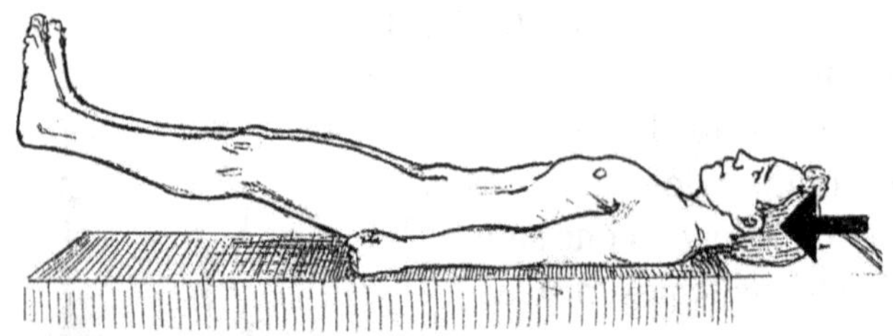

During the **CERVICAL COMPACTION TEST** the legs are more difficult to raise when the patient's cervical spine is compacted by the doctor's pedal pressure.

THE ARM FOSSA TEST

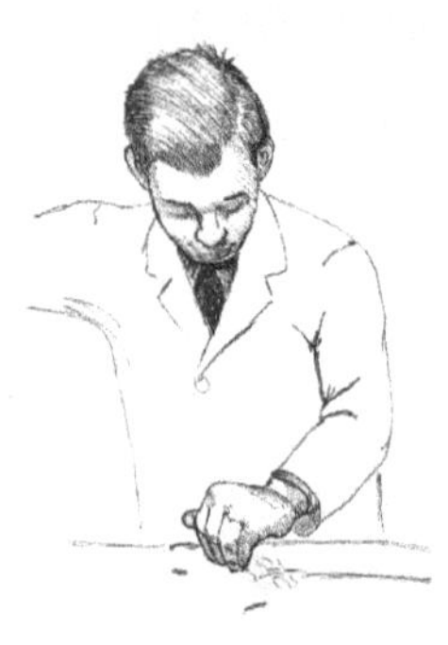

When one or more of the FOUR FOSSAE creates a weakness in the testing arm, there is a strong indicator for a CAT II.

Confirmation may be done by careful palpation along both INGUINAL ligaments, looking for a painful or sensitive nodule.

If the UPPER fossa is weak and/or painful, then the ilium is posterior of normal. The **KNEE ROTATES OUTWARDLY** and the **FOOT FLARES OUT.**

Remember the **UMS**: Upper Fossa, Medial Knee pain, Short Leg.

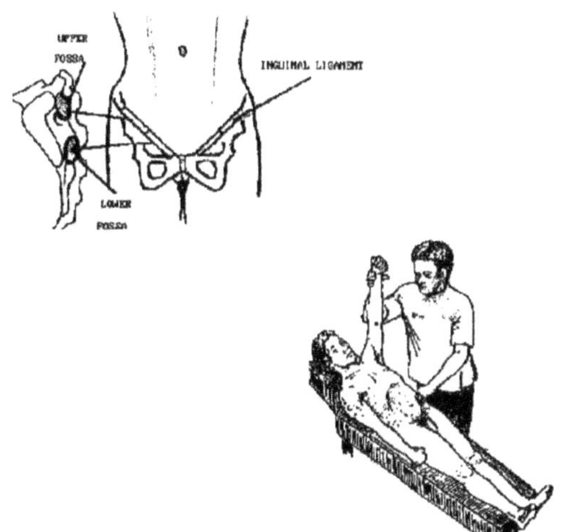

If the **LOWER Fossa** is involved, then the ilium is anterior of normal. The **KNEE ROTATES MEDIALLY** and the **FOOT PRONATES INWARDLY**.

Remember the **LLL**: Lower fossa, Lateral Knee pain, Long Leg.

If all of or most of the above are present, then the chances are pretty high that the patient is suffering from a Category II problem.

Before proceeding with the **BLOCKING Technique** adjust the patient with whatever adjustments are necessary. Since this is the first adjustment session, it is recommended to err on the side of under adjusting, especially if the patient has an acute CAT II problem. The blocking is a highly dynamic adjustment and deserves respect.

Blocking should be the last thing before sending the patient home; but always instruct the patient to walk for a while before sitting down especially in a car or bus.

5

CATEGORY II CORRECTION

The patient is lying prone, with the **PELVIC BOARD** placed beneath the pelvis. Make sure that it is well centered so there is room for the blocks to be placed clear of the edge. You have done the Fossa Test, which tells you that the Blocking is necessary today. The next thing you need to know is which is the physiological, or functional **SHORT LEG**.

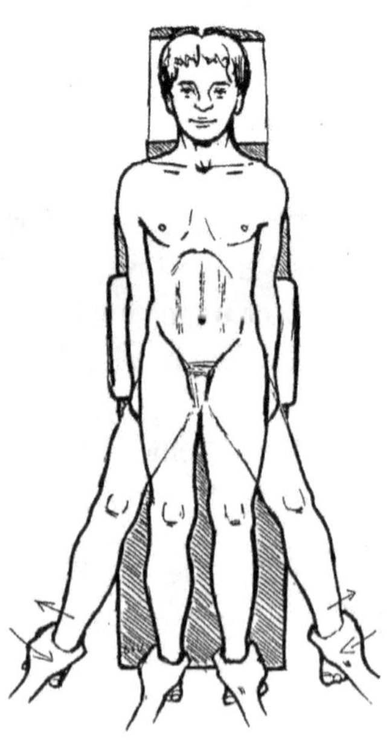

LEG LENGTH

Go to the feet and place one hand over each ankle, thumbs medially just below the medial malleoli. Compare the malleoli to see which one is higher, indicating a SHORT LEG.

Bring both legs apart and ask the patient to resist as you apply medial pressure. Then ask the patient to relax and bring the legs together again; recheck the leg lengths. If they have changed, then accept the last reading as correct.

If you are still in doubt about the SHORT LEG you can confirm it with a muscle test.

LEG LENGTH CONFIRMATION

Return to the patient's side and ask him to raise one arm as if for a fossa test. Test to determine the strong arm, then you may test either the long leg or the short leg, or both to be sure.

Place your hand just above the knee of the leg you are testing and exert a pedal stretch and retest the arm. Then place your hand below the knee and exert a cephalic pressure and retest the arm.

If the arm went weak with **lengthening** the leg (pedal/caudal stretch), then that was the **LONG LEG**. So then, of course if the arm went weak on **shortening** the leg (cephalic stretch) then it is the **SHORT LEG**. This test has come in very useful on many occasions. Additionally, it is about the only way to test in the presence of an amputee.

CATEGORY II BLOCKING

The patient is now lying relaxed (if possible) in the Supine position with the Pelvic Board beneath the pelvis. The Short leg side is established and recorded it in the patient's file.

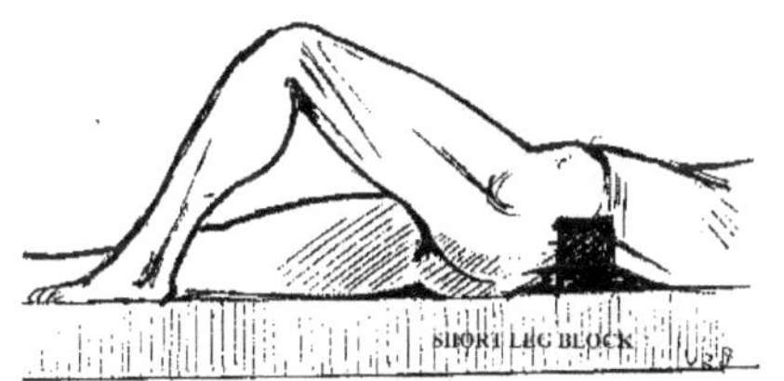

LEFT PSIS

Go to the side of the **SHORT LEG**. Ask the patient to slide his foot up the table so that the knee is bent to about 90°. Ask him to raise the pelvis on the **SHORT LEG** side by using the leg muscles.

Place the **UPPER BLOCK** under the **CREST** so that the rim of the crest bisects the block, and have the patient lower the pelvis onto the Block.

Now ask the patient to raise the LONG LEG Pelvis whilst you reach over and place the LOWER BLOCK beneath the ACETABULUM, with the leading edge pointing towards the end of the UPPER BLOCK. Make sure that the **PELVIS IS LEVEL WITH THE FLOOR.**

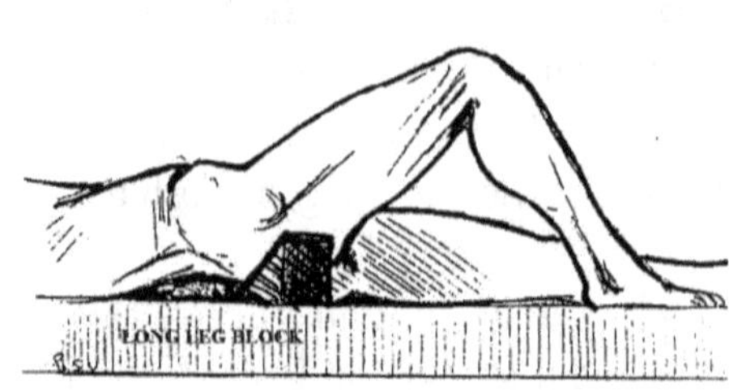

RIGHT ACETABULUM

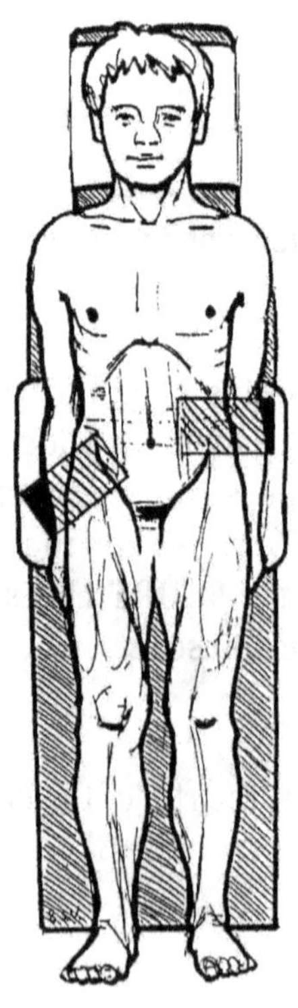

In this picture, the RIGHT LEG is the LONG LEG, and the LEFT LEG is the SHORT LEG.

The Patient is instructed to relax and keep the legs straight. This may be difficult but even at the expense of pain the legs must be straight.

The **Category II BLOCKING** is quite quick, from 30 seconds to a maximum of 2 minutes. The Fossa tests will tell you when you have achieved your objective.

THE FOUR WAY STRETCH

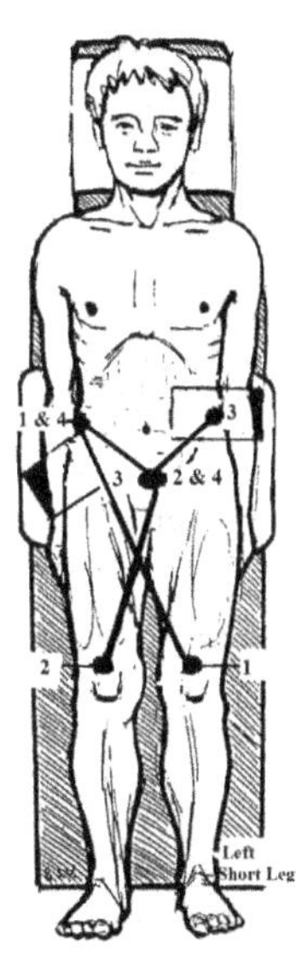

Moving quickly, contact the **LONG LEG SIDE** with the heel of the hand at the **ANTERIOR SPINE (ASIS)** and on the **SHORT LEG SIDE** with the flat hand just above the KNEE. Apply a stretch pressure against these two points.

Now bring the **TOP HAND** across to the **SHORT LEG SIDE PUBIS** and exchange the **LOWER HAND** to the **LONG LEG KNEE.** Stretch again.

The **TOP HAND** slides up to the **SHORT LEG ASIS** whilst **the LOWER HAND** moves up to contact the **LONG LEG PUBIS**. Stretch again.

Finally the hand on the **PUBIS** swaps sides to the **opposite PUBIS**, whilst the hand on the **ASIS** crosses to the **opposite ASIS**. Stretch once more.

Remember that with every Sacro-iliac distortion there must be a pubic distortion. This stretch helps to start the adjustment of the Sacro-iliac and also aids in the correction of the pubis involvement.

RETEST THE FOSSA: If still weak allow a little more time on the blocks. If strong, then the adjustment has been made. Ask the patient to remain relaxed whilst you gently lift one side just high enough to remove the block and lower gently. Be careful, a sudden drop can be painful. Then remove the other block in the same manner.

Ask the patient to walk around the room and thcn **RETEST ALL TIIE MIND LANGUAGE POINTS**. The patient should be instructed to walk briskly for a good fifteen to twenty minutes before sitting, especially in a car or bus. Also suggest that he walk each day to help to consolidate the adjustment.

THIS COVERS THE BASIC BLOCKING TECHNIQUE FOR CATEGORY II. BY LEARNING AND APPLYING THIS MUCH, THE DOCTOR WILL ALREADY BE DOING THE PATIENT A GREAT SERVICE. THERE IS MORE TO THE CATEGORY II COMPLEX PROCEDURE; THE NEXT CHAPTER COVERS ADDITIONAL STEPS. PERFECT THIS BASIC BLOCKING UNTIL YOU HAVE IT CHUNKED, THEN ADD TO THE CHUNKING AND EXPAND IT.

DISCUSSION

Now that you have been testing for Categories for a while, you must have noticed that a good percentage of cases show positive for a CAT II. Not all these cases had low back pain. Medical acceptance of any Sacral movement has been very slow in coming, but finally they have realized that what we have known for decades is in fact true: there is movement in the Sacro-iliac joint. *Gray's Anatomy* now reclassifies the SI joint as being a Synovial joint, as it contains synovial fluid and has detectable motion. The degree of motion is contained by the strong interosseous Anterior and Posterior Ligaments that bind the Sacrum to the Innominates.

The Category II problem starts when the Interosseous ligaments fail to limit the SI motion. The simple strain probably does not result in actual excess motion, but more by an awareness that the ligament is having difficulty trying to maintain that limitation and support. The Sprain then creates a laxity in ligamentous support, and so excess motion results. The Separation is of course self explanatory, causing great instability often to the extent that the patient is unable to take any weight on that SI joint.

The design of the SI joint is such that when there is laxity in the interosseous support ligaments the resultant displacement can only be Anterior.

Although the pelvis is surrounded by some of the most powerful muscles in the body, there are no muscles directly crossing the SI joint. The motion of the Sacrum is dictated by the movement of the innominates where the major muscles of locomotion within the torso and the legs are attached. The SOT blocking approach aims to replace the offending SI joint to a correct position, requiring it to be moved Posterior. The **Supine Blocking** procedure is very effective in this work and results in the minimum corrective trauma.

I am in no way detracting from other techniques that use the corrective adjustments to achieve the same purpose. The Blocking procedure would however be my choice for correcting a CAT II case.

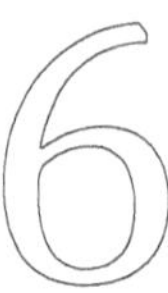

CATEGORY II FURTHER PROCEDURES

To expand upon Category II, understand the basic concept of the CAT II analysis and blocking procedure well before moving on. Do not try to do too much too soon. It is most important to do the right thing and to do it well.

THE CAT II BASIC CRANIAL TECHNIQUE

Because of the direct relationship between Sacral function and the skull (OCCIPUT), it would be remiss to ignore the distortions in the cranials that must be drawn into a CAT II problem.

CHECKING FOR POINT OF RESPIRATORY FIXATION

Prior to the Blocking, test one arm for strength as with the Fossa Test. Then ask the patient to take a full breath (INHALATION), pull the toes of both feet headward (cephalic) whilst tucking the chin in, thus forcing the face towards the feet. At the point of full INHALATION, with feet and head fully flexed, TEST THE ARM. If it remains strong, ask the patient to EXHALE completely, extend the feet and pull the head back. Once fully exhaled TEST THE ARM.

NOTE WHICH ONE WENT WEAK.

If the arm goes weak during INHALATION the CRANIAL ADJUSTMENT is made during EXHALATION. And contrastly, if the arm went weak on EXHALATION, then the CRANIAL ADJUSTMENT is made during INHALATION.

WEAKNESS during	FIXATION	ADJUSTMENT made on
INHALATON	Flexion	EXHALATION
EXHALATION	Extension	INHALATON

A WEAK ARM DURING EXHALATION

A weak arm during exhalation means that the Cranial fixation is caught in **EXTENSION** and cannot follow the INHALATION PHASE into FLEXION. The adjustment helps to restore the NORMAL RESPIRATORY MOTION.

ADJUSTMENT

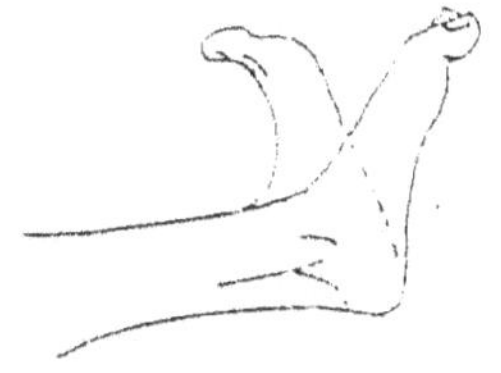

Instruct the patient to breathe in deeply and flex the toes towards the head. Then, as the patient breathes out extend the toes. The patient should get into a rhythm with the breathing and the toe movement. Go to the patient's head and cup one hand under the occiput. The other hand is the adjusting hand.

FIXED IN EXTENSION
(AT THE POINT OF FULL EXHALATION)

The arm went weak when the patient had exhaled. The Adjusting hand is placed palm down across the forehead, the fingers are divided so that two fingers are on either side of the nose. Contact the ZYGOMAS on either side. The heel of the hand contacts the FRONTAL BONE. As the patient breathes in, a gentle but firm PEDAL pressure is applied to the ZYGOMAS by the fingers, whilst the HEEL OF THE HAND keeps a firm pressure of the FRONTAL BONE. The OCCIPITAL hand merely HOLDS.

Time your rhythm by watching the patients' feet. As they are pulled towards you (Cephalically) make the adjustment. Relax when the feet start to move away from you (Pedally/Caudally).

FIXED IN FLEXION
(AT THE POINT OF FULL INHALATION)

The hands are in the same position but the pressure is the opposite. When the patient breathes OUT and the feet move away from you (PEDALLY/CAUDALLY), the fingers pull the ZYGOMAS up whilst the heel of the hand remains stationary. The OCCIPITAL HAND holds.

A SIMPLIFIED FORM OF CAT II CRANIAL ADJUSTING

As a great majority of patients seem to be fixed in FLEXION I, it is a useful technique to contact the OCCIPUT with one hand and the FRONTAL BONE with the other. The fingers of the FRONTAL HAND straddle the nose so that the second finger contacts one ORB whilst the third finger contacts the other ORB. As the patient EXHALES and the feet move PEDALLY a gentle but firm CEPHALIC pressure is exerted by the fingers as the hands try to move towards each other.

This is generally helping the CRANIUM to move into EXTENSION, which is the way it is trying to move during the EXHALATION phase of respiration.

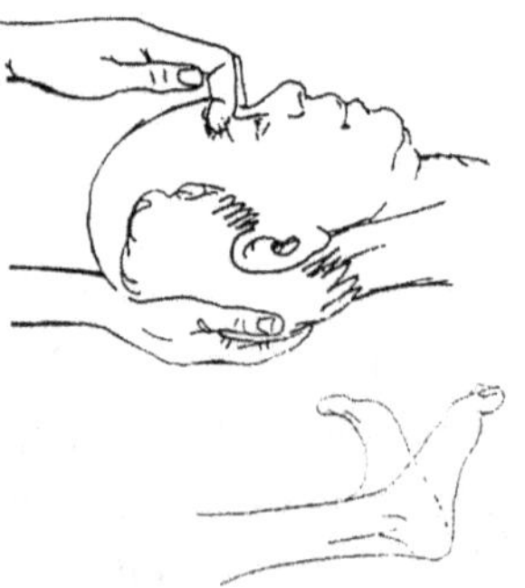

Often, the patient feels pain on one side or the other. With a little experience, the doctor will be able to feel a small nodule. When there is a painful nodule, exert just a little MORE pressure on that side.

A few Cycles is sufficient, ask the patient to relax again and then recheck the FOSSA TEST.

If all is well remove the blocks.

IT IS BEST TO WAIT UNTIL THE THIRD VISIT BEFORE DOING THE PSOAS CORRECTION. CORRECT THE PSOAS BEFORE BLOCKING.

THE PSOAS

Dr. de Jarnette teaches that the over-head/arm Psoas test is used to find the shorter arm indicating Psoas SPASM on the side of the short arm. The AK test can be used to find a WEAK Psoas. Both methods are described.

DE JARNETTE PSOAS TEST & CORRECTION

THE TEST

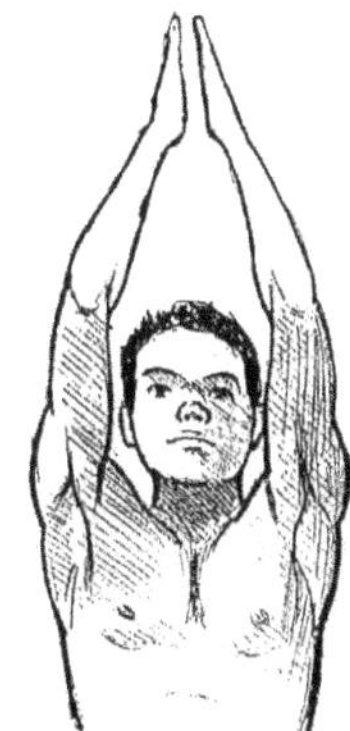

To test for a PSOAS involvement, ask the SUPINE patient to raise both hands above the head. The hands are turned inward with the fingers stretched. Grasp the wrists and exert a mild traction to see if one arm appears longer than the other.

The SHORTER ARM indicates PSOAS CONTRACTION OR SPASM.

THE PSOAS CORRECTION

Stand opposite the side of involvement. Ask the patient to bend the knee of the involved leg. Put the PEDAL hand beneath the patient's thigh and grasp the ANTERIOR SUPERIOR ILIAC SPINE.

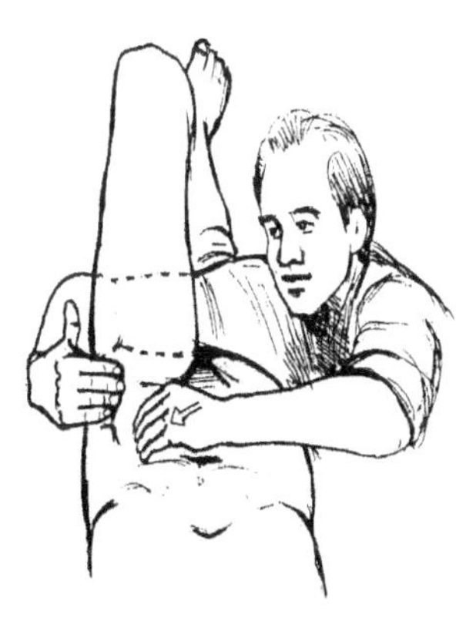

The CEPHALIC HAND is placed onto the abdomen just lateral to the umbilicus, pointing towards the inguinal region. Whilst holding an outward torsion on the ILIA, exert a gentle but firm pressure onto the PSOAS and ligaments in that region.

The hand is rotated to give a deep massage until some change is felt. Now retest the PSOAS. Go to the feet and recheck the LEG LENGTHS.

THE AK PSOAS TEST

The patient is in the SUPINE POSITION. Raise the leg to be tested about 45° from the table and ABDUCT it 45° from the center line.

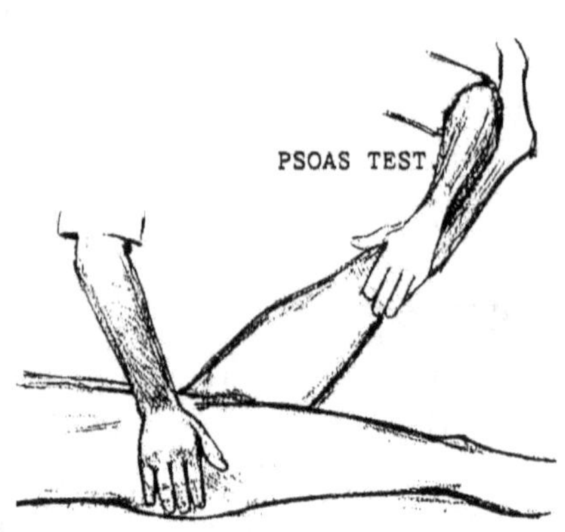

The leg remains straight during the test. Ask the patient to hold that position while you position the PEDAL/CAUDAL hand over the knee of the testing leg. The CEPHALIC hand is placed on the opposite ASIS.

Explain to the patient that you will put a pressure on the leg directed from ceiling to floor at a 45° angle towards you (the doctor). The patient should resist towards the ceiling at 45° away from you.

Test both legs in this manner and look for a weak response.

The weaker leg indicates a weak PSOAS and this is the one to STIMULATE.

If the patient is still in pain and/or unable to raise a straight leg, then the AK Psoas Test may be difficult to perform. So, the ARM TEST can still be used to indicate a weak psoas; the weak psoas is on the side of the LONGER ARM.

If the ARM TEST showed one arm short and the LEG TEST did not show a weakness, then clearly the CONTRACTED PSOAS would be the one to correct. However, if there is a weakness in the LEG (AK) test, then the following correction for a weak psoas would be indicated.

THE CORRECTION FOR A WEAK PSOAS

Stand opposite the side being corrected. Ask the patient to bend the knee on the side to be corrected. Support the knee with your PEDAL/CAUDAL HAND, pulling it slightly towards you.

Place the tips of your fingers into the lower abdomen just lateral to the umbilicus on the treatment side. As your fingers go in to find the PSOAS, draw the knee a little more towards you.

The correction is a gentle but firm caressing movement along the PSOAS. Continue this for a few minutes and then RETEST THE PSOAS. If you have done it correctly you will see a difference.

If the Psoas Correction is indicated, perform the correction prior to the Blocking.

BALANCING THE LEG LENGTHS

BLOCKING does not balance the LEG LENGTHS in the CAT II. Once the Blocking has done its work and the patient is becoming pain free (probably about the third visit) it is time to balance the leg length deficiency. THIS CAN BE PERFORMED AFTER THE BLOCKS HAVE BEEN REMOVED.

SHORT LEG TECHNIQUE

Stand on the SHORT LEG SIDE. Flex the knee of the SHORT LEG, holding it by the knee and the ankle. With the knee at about a 90° angle, push the knee MEDIALLY and keep the medial pressure as you lower the leg to the table again.

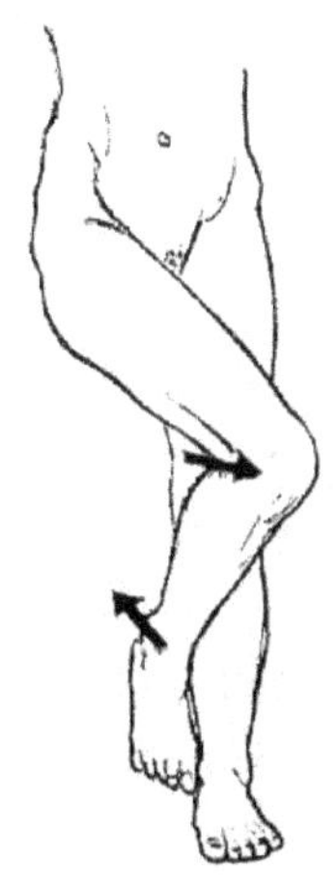

LONG LEG TECHNIQUE

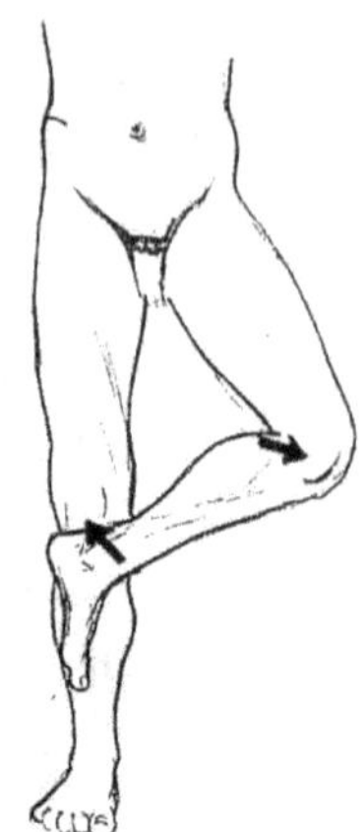

Still standing on the SHORT LEG SIDE, flex the LONG LEG, again holding the knee and the ankle. The ankle is held slightly lateral to the short leg.

The knee hand presses the knee LATERALLY. The pressure is held as the ankle is slid down the table until the leg returns to the straight position.

LUMBAR ADJUSTMENTS IN THE CATEGORY II COMPLEX

As the CAT II begins to stabilize the Lumbar spine may be in need of adjustment. It is important to allow the Sacro-iliac Joint to begin the healing process before exerting anything more than the lightest adjustment. This is especially true in the Separation and Sprain cases. When you feel that it is prudent to make an adjustment, recheck the Fossa for weakness after you have made the adjustment, if it became weak, then Block as the last thing of the session.

THE ACETABULAR BELT

Sometimes it will be necessary to give the Sacra-iliac a little support while it is regaining strength. This is especially true where a SEPARATION has occurred and also true where the same FOSSA is weak on the third visit.

The patient should wear the belt for four or five days, day and night. It can be removed for washing, but suggest that the patient take a shower rather than a sit-down bath while the belt is off. After wearing the belt for four or five days consistently, the patient may gradually remove it for longer periods. As sleeping is always a bad time for CAT II patients, it may be necessary for a while to keep the belt on at night (it may be loosened a bit), whilst removing it for periods during the day. It could well be six to twelve weeks before the patient can be completely weaned of the belt.

ULTRA-SOUND

When there has been SEPARATION, ULTRA-SOUND is most effective for helping to dry out the Inter-osseous ligament.

ICE

During the acute phase of a SPRAIN, ICE helps to reduce the inflammatory process. It should be applied at the pain site with a towel placed over the skin and the ice bag on top of the towel. The maximum time for each application is ten minutes. After the icing the patient should walk around a little. Icing followed by walking can be done several times a day.

HEAT

Once the acute phase is over and healing is taking place, HEAT can be applied to facilitate healing.

THE TRAPEZIUS

The Trapezius analysis and adjustive technique is not essentially a Category associated technique, as it is appropriate whenever there are muscle, tendon or joint pains. However, experience has shown that it is especially helpful in association with the Category II (and the Occipital Technique is more appropriate in association with Category I).

As a follow-up procedure or as a general check-up procedure the Trapezius technique comes into its own. By careful palpation of the Trapezius muscle, as it crosses the shoulders, the experienced practitioner can identify a vertebral area that is in mechanical distress. The subluxation that needs adjusting is located by identifying the specific vertebra with palpation of the surrounding muscle. The Thoracic and Lumbar vertebrae are more intimately involved in the Trapezius complex than the Cervicals.

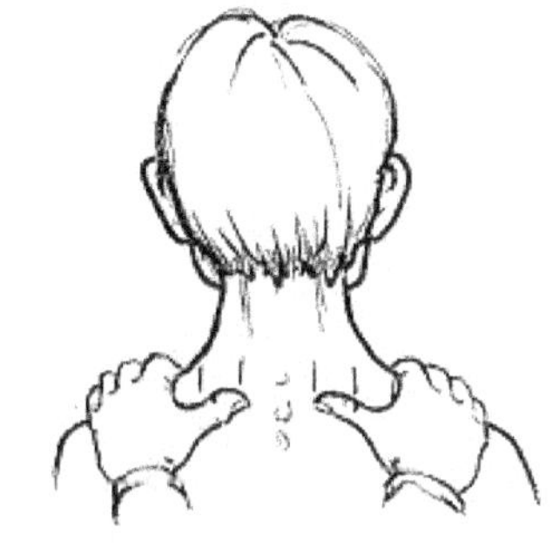

CATEGORY II FURTHER PROCEDURES

The Trapezius taut and tender fiber identifies a FAMILY of vertebrae with members in the Cervical, Thoracic and Lumbar spine. By examining the individual members of that family the Chiropractor discovers the offending vertebra and adjusts it.

As soon as the patient is sufficiently recovered to be comfortable, it is time to check the Trapezius and adjust accordingly. This may be the second or third visit.

While the patient is lying PRONE, palpate along a line between the ACROMIOCLAVICULAR NOTCH and the lateral edge of the body of the 1st THORACIC VERTEBRA (T1).

This imaginary line is slightly bow-shaped with the arch of the bow pointing downwards.

This line is divided into seven equal parts with the first being just medial to the ACROMIOCLAVICULAR NOTCH and the last being the final fleshy part before encountering the spinous process of T1.

The palpating is directed to find a tight and raised band or bands of the Trapezius muscle which when found will lead you to a vertebra or vertebrae that are part of a musculo-skeletal distortion and need adjusting.

The Trapezius Analytical Chart can assist with identifying the vertebra or vertebrae that are correlated with the taut or tender Trapezius zone.

TRAPEZIUS ANALYTICAL CHARTS

Trapezius Line	7	6	5	4	3	2	1
Thoracic							
T1							1
T2							1
T3						2	
T4					3		
T5					3		
T6				4			
T7			5				
T8		6					
T9	7						
T10							1
T11						2	
T12						2	
Lumbar							
L1					3		
L2				4			
L3			5				
L4		6					
L5	7						

The adjustment is done by a flat hand, little finger, nail point #1 contact. The thrust is superior allowing for laterality. The action is a quick, lifting SUPERIOR scoop. This subluxation is not involved in a respiratory cycle, so just ask the patient to breathe in and let the air out to gain relaxation.

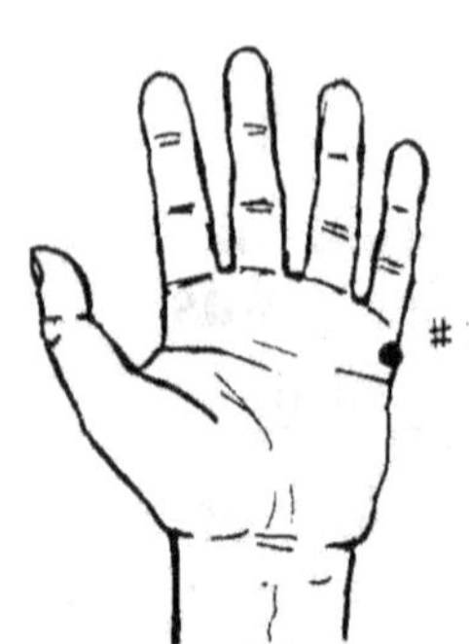

The painful fibers may be unilateral or bilateral, single or multiple, so make a thorough examination and do not stop as soon as you find *one*.

THE FEET

A STABLE PELVIS REQUIRES A STABLE ARCH SUPPORT (and vice versa). A weakened pelvis will have a detrimental effect on the knees, ankles and the arches of the feet. It is just as true to say that weakened arches will have a detrimental effect on the knees, pelvis and so also the remainder of the spine, just as a weakened pelvis affects the entire spine above.

Examination of the arches and the knees are an important part of the examination. A badly weakened arch is very difficult to repair. Where the ligamenture of the foot has lost its supportive strength, no amount of exercises can return it to a normal arch.

If the arch is seriously involved, the Chiropractor must advise the patient that the CAT II problem cannot be stabilized for long unless a corrective ORTHOTIC is provided.

When examining the feet, stand the patient with the feet parallel, just a few inches apart.

Look at the way the feet lie, are the arches intact?
Are the arches equal?
Look at the Calcanei, are they upright or do they angle?
Look at the line of the big toe, is it straight or angled?
Are the toes flat or drawn up?
The patella SHOULD point the same way the feet point, do they?
Are the knees too close or too far apart?

As a rule, the dropped arch will cause the calcaneous to appear angled. The big toe will tend to angle laterally because, as the Cuneiforms and the Navicular flatten and swing medially, the first Metatarsal rotates. This is the beginning of the BUNION.

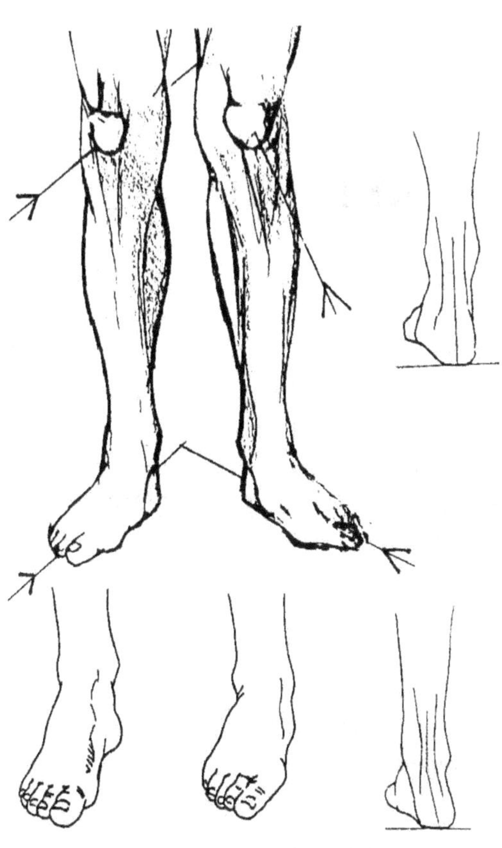

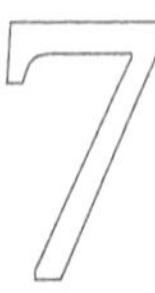

CATEGORY II REHABILITATION

The acute or severe CAT II must be considered as a serious injury that requires healing time once the Sacra-iliac separation, sprain, or strain has been reduced by blocking. There are no muscles directly involved in the Sacra-iliac Joint as the movement in the joint is highly limited and controlled indirectly by the movement and positioning of the innominates that have major muscle connections with the trunk and legs.

Once the patient has reached the point where no further blocking is necessary, as determined by the FOSSA TEST, the patient must be cautioned that the SI joint is still in a highly vulnerable state, and that stretching, twisting, lifting or prolonged awkward positions can upset it. The legs should not be crossed when sitting and care should be taken whilst getting up from a chair.

The best form of exercise is walking and the patient should be advised to go for a brisk walk every day.

A USEFUL HOME EXERCISE

One exercise that can help to tighten up the area is done lying SUPINE on a smooth surface. The patient needs someone to help with this exercise.

The patient draws both legs up so that the knees are bent to an angle less than 90°.

The feet remain on the floor or smooth surface. The helper contacts both knees with a hand supporting each knee from the medial surface.

The knees are held wide apart at first. The patient then lowers the legs by sliding the heels along the floor or smooth surface, whilst bringing the knees together against the helper's resistance (the resistance should be just enough to make it a little difficult but not impossible) to end up with the legs flat and the knees together.

Now the reverse is done, with the helper resisting with a medial pressure as the patient bends the knees by sliding the feet upwards the buttocks and moving the knees apart.

This is an exercise for home use and can be done two or three times a day, starting with a few cycles with light helper pressure, and increasing both cycles and the pressure as more strength is acquired.

THE FIRST SIX WEEKS

The CAT II should be checked periodically through the first six weeks to make sure that it holds.

The CAT II is a time bomb that can go-off at anytime, so the CAT II patient should be carefully checked each time he comes back for a check-up.

Once the doctor is sure that the CAT II is stable, the patient is checked for CAT I to end up with a PHYSIOLOGICAL CAT I PATIENT.

It may be necessary to BLOCK a patient in the prone position, especially when there is a mixture of CAT II and CAT III. The Mind Language Test will indicate when this is necessary. However, if there is some doubt about the stability of the CAT II, which could be weakened during the CAT III blocking, there is a way of solving this.

A simple canvas or leather belt can be placed around the patient's pelvis. The belt will help to support the weight-bearing part of the SI Joint during the prone CAT III blocking.

THE TMJ

I will only attempt to introduce the TMJ, but it is a very important part of the CAT II patient care, and needs more study to understand.

Chronic loss of weight bearing integrity in the SI Joint creates distortion in the relationship between the Occiput and the Temporals. The TMJ articulates with the Temporal bones and so any distortion will cause an uneven seating of the TMJ in the Temporo-mandibular fossa, malocclusion of the teeth will be a logical result.

If the situation remains for some time the patient may experience clicking in the jaw. Eventually the TM disc can be damaged and arthritic changes take place in the joint.

Bruxism (grinding the teeth) is often experienced. Usually the spouse will be the one to identify the bruxism, as the sound of someone grinding his or her teeth can be very annoying.

Suffice it at this point to recognize the TMJ as a cousin of the CAT II problem, and when the doctor becomes experienced with using SOT this is a very useful area for further study. Be prepared and willing to work in association with a dentist on these cases. A chronic TMJ problem, once resolved still requires dental care to correct the bite.

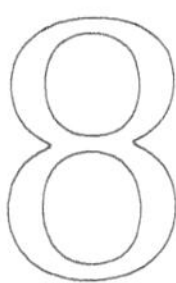

CATEGORY III

Through testing, it is revealed that the patient has a CATEGORY III problem.

CASE HISTORY FINDINGS

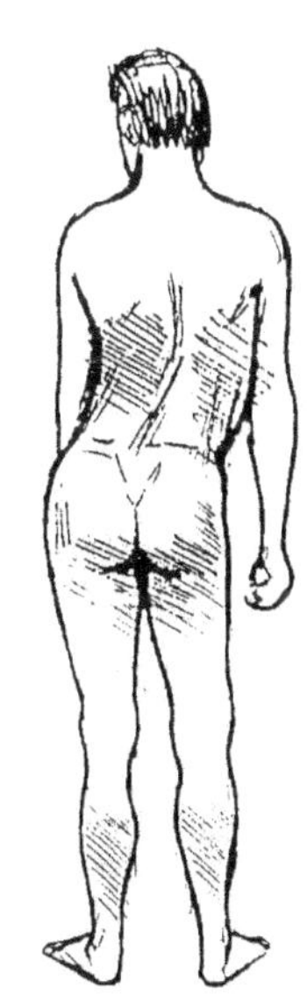

The patient complained of severe SCIATICA, with or without lumbar pain.

The true Sciatic pain is from the Buttocks down the posterior thigh and calf.

The onset could have been either gradual or sudden.

The pain is usually worse on weight bearing and especially walking.

Sitting can also be extremely uncomfortable.

Coughing or sneezing exacerbates the condition.

There is often previous history of back pain.

AT THE PLUMB LINE: The patient cannot stand straight. There is a marked **ANTALGIC LEAN**. The lean may be either towards the side of sciatica or away from it; **NOTE WHICH.** The pelvis is intact; there is no lateral sway and no AP sway.

NOTE: NOT ALL CAT III's HAVE THE ANTALGIC LEAN OR SCIATICA SO KEEP AN OPEN MIND. NEVER JUMP TO CONCLUSIONS.

MIND LANGUAGE

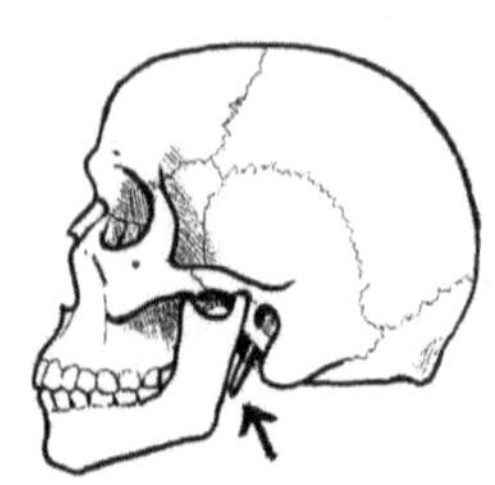

A strong arm goes weak when the finger contacted the STYLOID PROCESS. Weakness on contacting the mammilary process of the lumbar vertebrae also indicates CAT III.

THE ARM FOSSA TEST is NEGATIVE.

THE LEG RAISING TEST is probably difficult to assess because of pain. If it is possible, it would show negative.

THE CERVICAL COMPACTION TEST would also be difficult to assess.

NEUROLOGICAL TESTS would help to isolate the level of involvement and type of dysfunction.

Lasegue, Patella and Achilles reflexes would be relevant.

TEST FOR BIG TOE STRENGTH: a weakness indicates L4 involvement.

ROCKING TEST: the patient tries to rock backward and forward, if unable to keep balance, a NUCLEUS PULPOSUS HERNIATION is suspect.

PSOAS: the patient unable to raise one bent knee. Also pain on sitting or walking may indicate PSOAS involvement.

The classic CAT III is fairly easy to spot, but there are many borderline cases that are not so easy to distinguish from the CAT I or CAT II, so evaluate each test carefully.

TO BLOCK A CAT III AS A CAT II OR VICE VERSA IS TO COURT DISASTER

After the evaluation, if you are sure that the patient is suffering from a CAT III problem, we can go on to the SOT BLOCKING TECHNIQUE.

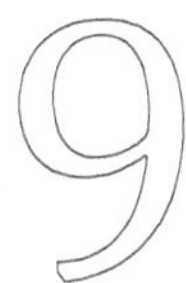

CATEGORY III DEFINED

The presenting **CATEGORY III** is not usually the result of a recent trauma, but more often the result or prolonged stress, probably in the presence of an uncorrected CAT I or II complex, or previous trauma resulting in a loss of disc integrity.

The human **DISC** is a very strong structure. It is made up of a viscous NUCLEUS PULPOSUS encased in a multilayered **ANNULUS FIBROSIS.**

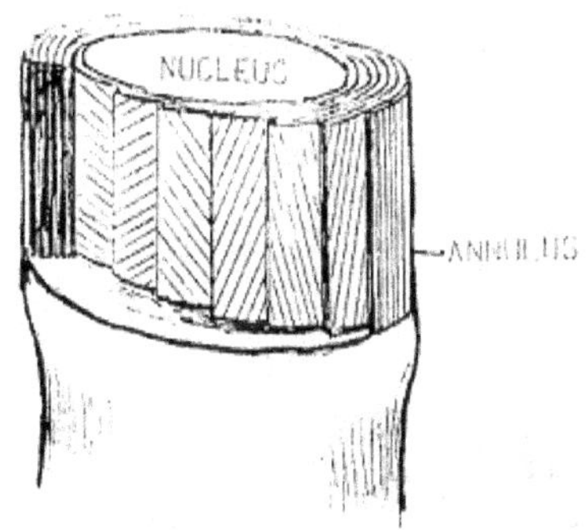

The layers of the **ANNULUS** start at the **NUCLEUS** with fibers that are almost horizontal.

Each onion-like layer becomes more angled, until the outer layer is almost vertical. This configuration makes for a very strong Disc, still allowing for movement and shock absorption.

When the PELVIS becomes impaired it throws a great deal of stress into the **LUMBAR SPINE**, eventually bringing about a breakdown in the integrity or the **ANNULUS**. This can lead to either **FRAGMENTATION of the ANNULUS**, or a shift in the position of the **NUCLEAR SUBSTANCE**, which results in a **BULGING**.

Similarly weight-bearing trauma, especially where there is simultaneous rotation can cause disc injury. Either of these situations can lead to neurological distress due to cord or nerve root pressure.

OTHER CAUSES OF THE CAT III

LUMBAR SUBLUXATION with occlusion at the foramen, with nerve root compression or traction; either as a rotation or tippage subluxation.

Contraction of the PSOAS muscle pulling on one of the discs. The PSOAS originates in part from the ANNULUS FIBROSIS of the Lumbar vertebrae.

An elongation of the PIRIFORMIS muscle can trap the SCIATIC NERVE.

These causes are differentiated later.

THE ANTALGIC LEAN

The antalgic lean so common in the CAT III situation is the body's attempt to minimize the effects of the disc's contact with the spinal cord or nerve root.

ANTALGIC LEAN AWAY FROM SCIATIC LEG

If the Antalgic lean is **away from** the SCIATIC LEG, it indicates a FRAGMENTATION or protrusion of the ANNULUS caused by the wedging of the disc material between two vertebrae. The disc encroachment is on the thin side of the wedge.

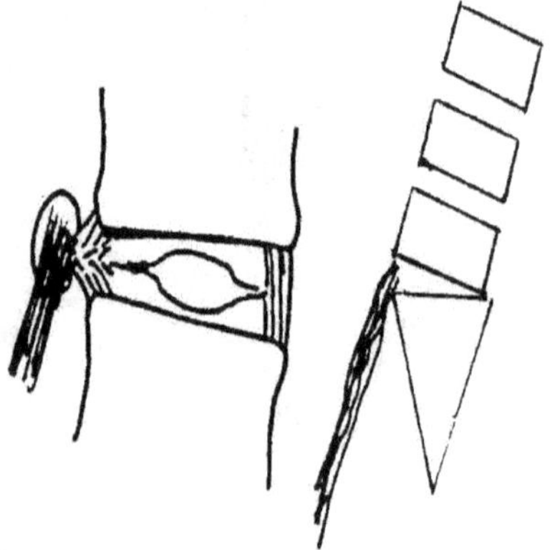

The body is trying to minimize the wedge, and pulls the lumbar spine to the opposite side.

ANTALGIC LEAN TOWARDS SCIATIC LEG

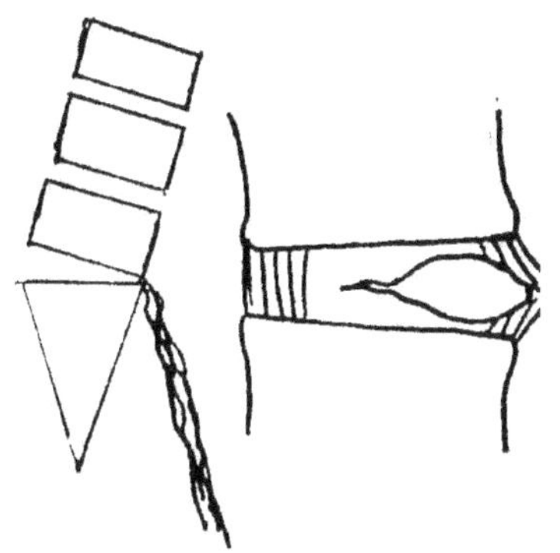

When the Antalgic lean is **towards** the side of SCIATIC INVOLVEMENT, then there is a BULGING of the NUCLEUS on the open side of a wedge.

The body is trying to minimize the wedge.

10

CATEGORY III CORRECTION

The CATEGORY III CORRECTION is non-invasive, and therefore very safe, way of handling a disc problem. The positioning of the blocks allows for a pain-free position to allow the lumbar spine a chance to relax and decrease the tension. The gradual relaxing of the lumbar spine in this position also allows for a repositioning of the offending structures.

THE CATEGORY III CORRECTION

It is time to get on and help this poor suffering patient. Do not try to adjust this patient, especially if he is leaning TOWARDS the side of SCIATICA. The kindest and most worthwhile thing you can do for the patient is to get him comfortably onto the BLOCKS.

POSITIONING

The patient is PRONE with the PELVIC BOARD UNDER THE PELVIS. Allow the patient time to become relaxed. It can take a little time so don't hurry the patient. Check the leg lengths. Grasp both ankles with the thumbs across the ACHILLES TENDONS just superior to the CALCANEOUS. **Compare the MEDIAL MALLEOLI and RECORD THE SIDE OF THE SHORT LEG.**

Have the patient hold the top of the table and resist whilst the doctor pulls both legs firmly but gently. Compare the MEDIAL MALLEOLI. RECORD THE SIDE OF THE SHORT LEG. IF THERE IS A DIFFERENCE BETWEEN THE FIRST AND SECOND READING TAKE THE SECOND

READING AND NOTE THE FACT IN YOUR RECORDS. ON SUBSEQUENT VISITS TAKE THE SAME READING.

Cat III Blocking Right Short Leg

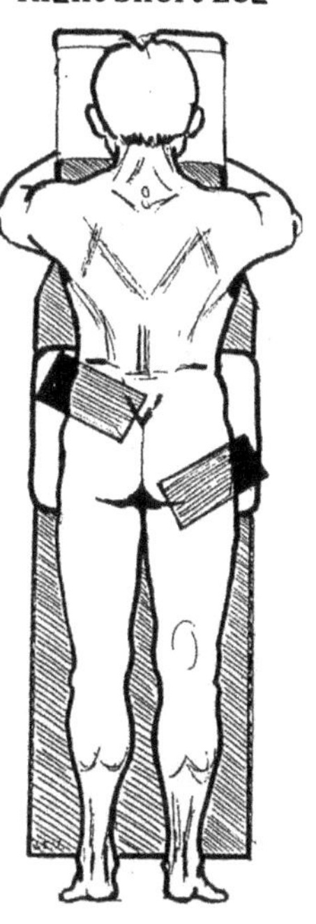

Stand on the LONG LEG SIDE. Reach over and raise the pelvis on the SHORT LEG SIDE. Insert a block under the ACETABULUM angled about 45° towards the feet.

Then raise the pelvis on the LONG LEG SIDE and insert the block under the ANTERIOR ILIAC CREST. Also angled 45° towards the feet.

ENSURE THE PELVIS IS LEVEL.

Go to the patient's feet again and instruct the patient to hold the top of the table and resist the doctor's pull with his arms whilst trying to relax the rest of the body as much as possible.

Grasp the SCIATIC LEG with both hands and exert a firm smooth traction, making sure the patient is resisting enough to maintain his position on the blocks.

After a few seconds gradually release the pull and let the patient relax.

NOTE: Once the SHORT LEG is established, it will remain THE SHORT LEG for this patient, so make sure to have the CORRECT SHORT LEG.

ADJUSTING THE BLOCK POSITION

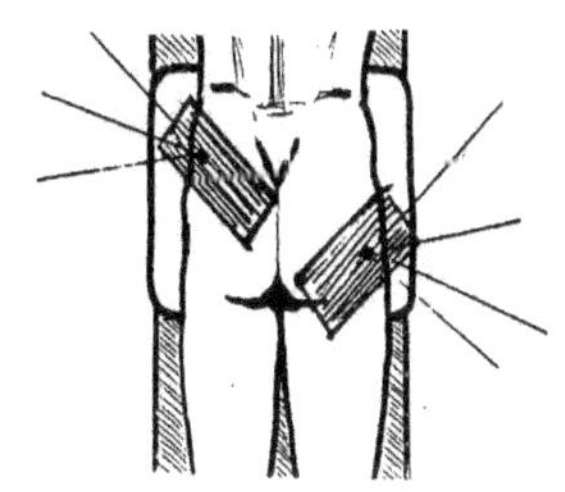

After a minute inquire from the patient whether the pain is less. If it is, then leave him alone for a while.

When you are more confident you may leave the patient who has settled and go to see another patient.

If the pain does not subside after a minute or two, change the angle of the LOWER block.

Wait for a minute to see if the pain diminishes. If it does not, keep adjusting the angle of the blocks, giving a minute to see the result - until the correct positioning is found. If no angle makes a difference, return the lower block to the original position and then adjust the UPPER block.

One method of testing for the correct position of the blocks is to find the pain area in the calf and the buttock. Retest them after each movement of the blocks. If a particular positioning of the blocks reduces the pain areas it is the correct positions for the blocks to remain in for the treatment.

The buttock pain is usually found just above the DOLLAR sign (Explained in CAT I).

Once a comfortable position is found, leave the patient to relax.

At the end of the blocking time, check the patient to see if the muscles seem more relaxed. Do not prod, but instead observe.

The Cough Test followed by the SB + or SB – leg traction technique can be used at this point, but only if a cough test can be done without causing distress. These are covered in detail under CAT I.

There are other procedures that can be done, depending on the nature or the CAT III problem. The procedures are covered next, with the explanation of the different CAT III types.

TIPPAGE OR ROTATION

The LUMBAR vertebrae can either TIP or ROTATE and cause traction or compression of the nerve roots or the cord.

TIPPING is more likely when there are SAGITTAL FACETS as they would restrict rotation but allow the lateral tipping motion. Tipping can cause traction of the nerve root on the open side of the wedge.

ROTATION is more likely when there are CORONAL FACETS as the rotary motion is less impaired but tipping is restricted.

Both TIPPAGE and ROTATION can involve either the NUCLEUS PULPOSUS or the ANNULUS.

The examination must determine the mechanics involved as well as the nature of the disc damage. The rule of thumb is if the patient leans towards the sciatic leg, the nucleus pulposus is involved.

TIPPAGE WITH NERVE ROOT TRACTION

This is a subluxation where the vertebra has tipped and causes a protrusion of the ANNULUS that causes Foraminal Nerve Root Traction.

The ANTALGIC LEAN will be towards the side OPPOSITE the sciatic involvement.

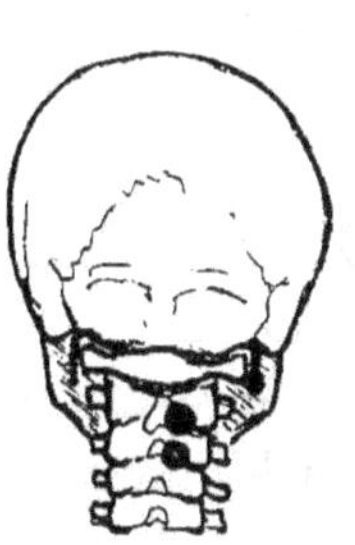

PAIN PATTERNS

5th Lumbar - Pain on STYLOID on the side of LUMBAR INFERIORITY.

4th Lumbar - Pain on lateral aspect of the AXIS SPINOUS on the side of LUMBAR INFERIORITY.

3rd Lumbar - Pain on the lateral aspect of the C3 SPINOUS on the side of LUMBAR INFERIORITY.

This subluxation will respond to manual adjustment if you feel it is preferable, but remember **ALWAYS PLACE THE PATIENT WITH THE PAIN SIDE DOWN.**

The Adjustment should reduce the tippage.

TIPPAGE WITH NUCLEUS BULGE

Degeneration and Prolapse of the disc material produces cord and/or nerve root pressure.

Where there is a lateral protrusion of the NUCLEUS PULPOSUS causing sciatica, the ANTALGIC LEAN will be TOWARDS the side of SCIATICA.

PAIN PATTERN

There will usually be NO Styloid or Cervical pain, but where there is it will be BILATERAL.

If there is Styloid or Cervical pain check the PSOAS and PIRIFORMIS. Remember the Psoas is attached to Lumbar discs and can be the cause of disc involvement.

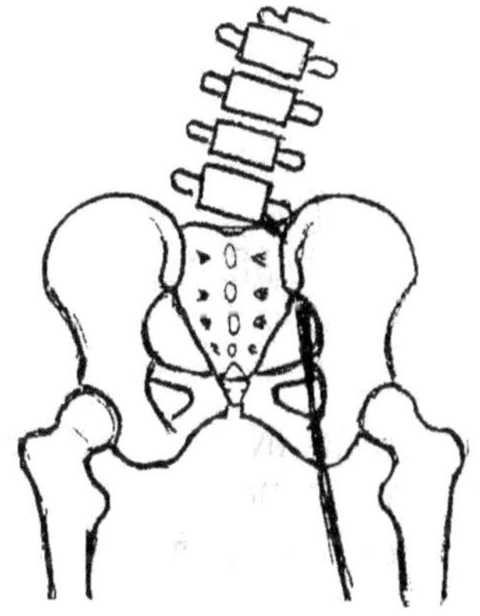

No Adjustment should be given where there is a disc bulge. The blocks are the method of choice. The prognosis for an antalgic lean on the side of sciatica is not good, so monitor it well. Surgery may be necessary.

ROTATION SUBLUXATION

The Rotation subluxation is more likely when the facets are angled more towards the CORONAL plane. There may be an antalgic lean, either towards or away from the SCIATIC LEG.

The rules are the same. If the LEAN is TOWARDS the SCIATICA it means there is a NUCLEAR BULGE. It is more likely that there will be a RAINBOW CURVATURE rather than a lean.

The rule here is if the spinous rotates away from the side of sciatica there is disc involvement. If it rotates towards the sciatic side then the nerve root is compressed.

ROTATION WITH NERVE ROOT COMPRESSION

The RAINBOW CURVATURE is easier to see with the aid of a PLUMB LINE.

THE SPINOUS WILL BE ROTATED TOWARDS THE SIDE OF SCIATICA.

PAIN PATTERN

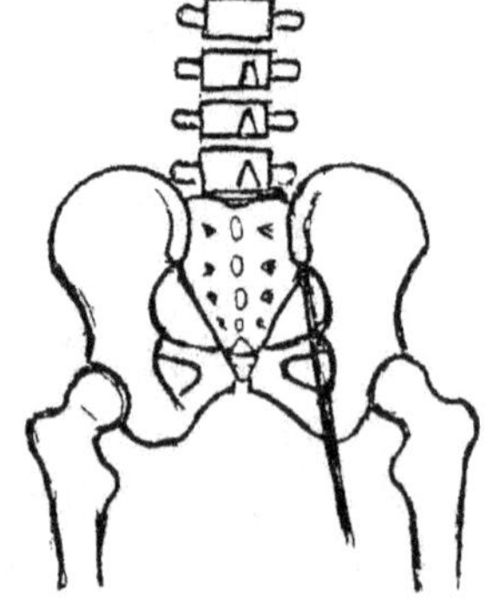

5th Lumbar - Pain on the ATLAS TRANSVERSE on side of SPINOUS ROTATION.

4th Lumbar - Pain on the AXIS TRANSVERSE on side of SPINOUS ROTATION.

3rd Lumbar - Pain on 3C TRANSVERSE on side of SPINOUS ROTATION.

When there is ROTATION the best means of correcting it following the blocking is by use of the ORTHOPEDIC BLOCK. (Explained on a later page.)

MANUAL CORRECTION CAN BE DONE, BUT DO NOT ROTATE THE SPINE AS IN THE LUMBAR ROLL. SECURE THE PELVIS AND MERELY ROTATE THE OFFENDING VERTEBRA.

MAKE SURE THAT THE **PAIN SIDE IS DOWN**.

ROTATION WITH DISC DEGENERATION AND PROLAPSE

Degeneration and Prolapse of the disc material produces cord and/or nerve root pressure.

Where there is a lateral protrusion of the Nucleus Pulposus causing Sciatica, the ANTALGIC LEAN will be TOWARDS the side of Sciatica in an attempt to minimize the protrusion.

In the true ROTATION, however, there is more often a RAINBOW CURVATURE with the SPINOUS ROTATION AWAY FROM THE SIDE OF SCIATICA.

DO NOT USE MANUAL CORRECTION IN THE PRESENCE OF A DISC INVOLVEMENT. The scissors type action of the Lumbar Roll can cause further damage to the disc. This is malpractice country so stay clear. It is possible that the CAT III problem seen with this came about by injudicious lumbar rolls in the past.

PAIN PATTERN

Usually with DISC INVOLVEMENT in a ROTATION SUBLUXATION there is NO STYLOID or CERVICAL PAIN. If there is pain it will be bilateral:

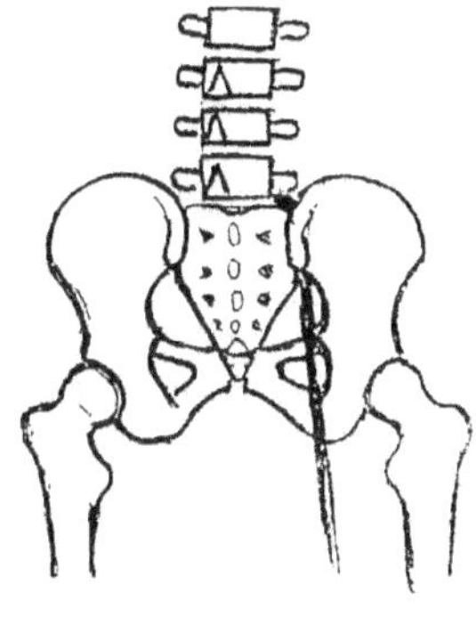

5th Lumbar - BOTH atlas transverses.
4th Lumbar - BOTH axis transverses.
3rd Lumbar - BOTH C3 transverses.

The ORTHOPEDIC BLOCK can also be used following CAT III Blocking.

THE ORTHOPEDIC BLOCK

The object is to elevate one side of the pelvis in such a way as to encourage the rotated vertebra to correct itself.

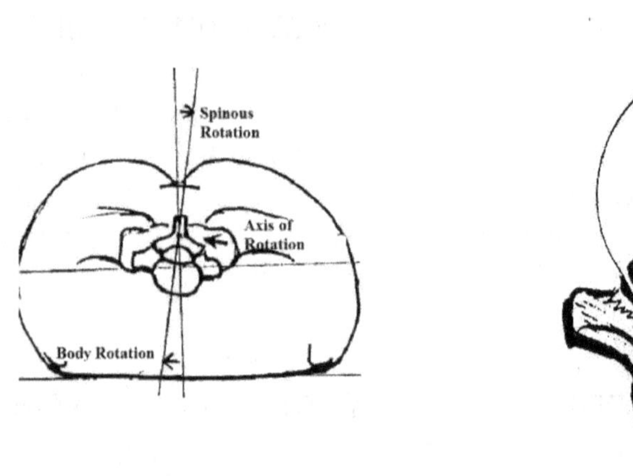

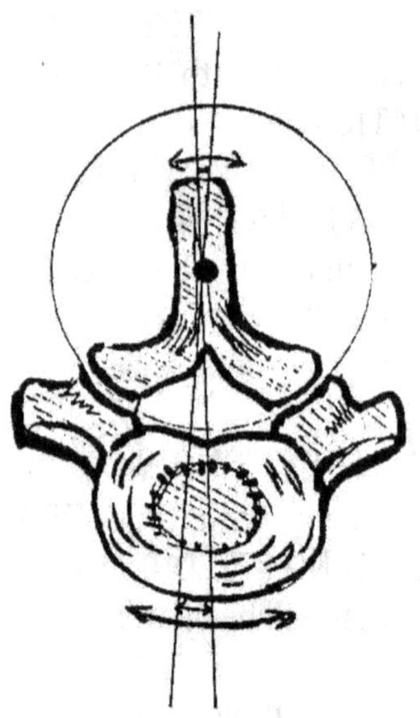

The high side is on the side away from the spinous process rotation. This puts the body of the vertebra on the high side. Gravity will exert its force on the body so that as it swings towards the floor the spinous will swing up, seeming to move up-hill.

Once the CAT III BLOCKING is almost complete, the BLOCK ON THE SIDE OF SPINOUS ROTATION is removed. The remaining block can be rotated to face directly across the pelvis.

With the block raising the pelvis so that the spinous is towards the Low side it will rotate UPHILL. The BODY will be encouraged to swing DOWNHILL.

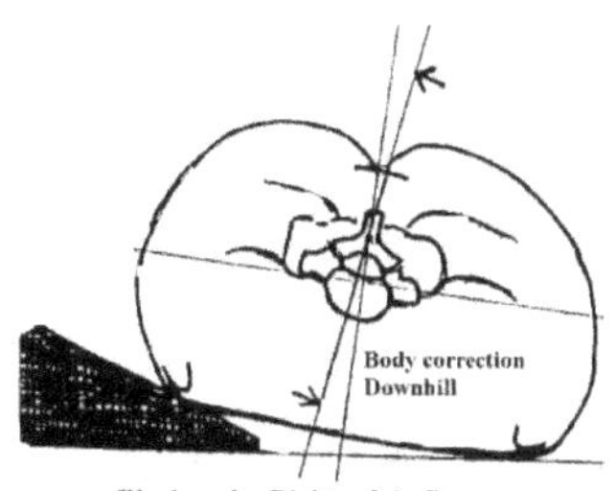

Block under Right pelvis. Prone

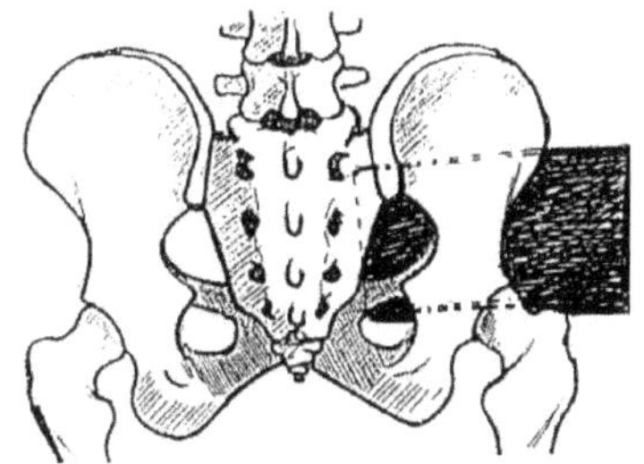

The foot on the LOW SIDE is raised with knee bent so that the heel is brought as close to the buttock as possible. A slight rhythmic pressure can be applied to both the foot and the spinous process to help the correction,

This may not always be possible because of pain, so use your judgment.

LEAVE THE PATIENT ON THE ORTHOPEDIC BLOCK FOR A FURTHER FEW MINUTES.

ANTERIOR LUMBAR SYNDROME OR SPONDYLOLISTHESIS

Where there is BILATERAL SCIATICA with or without ANTALGIC LEAN look for the ANTERIOR LUMBAR or the SPONDYLOLISTHESIS.

PAIN PATERNS

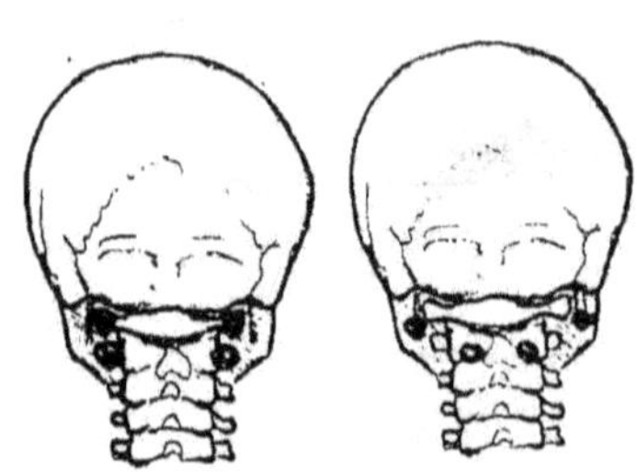

ANTALGIC LEAN: BOTH STYLOIDS and both sides of the AXIS SPINOUS.

WITHOUT LEAN: BOTH ATLAS TRANSVERSES and BOTH AXIS TRANSVERSES.

The PRONE BLOCKING would be indicated.

THE ANTERIOR LUMBAR TECHNIQUE

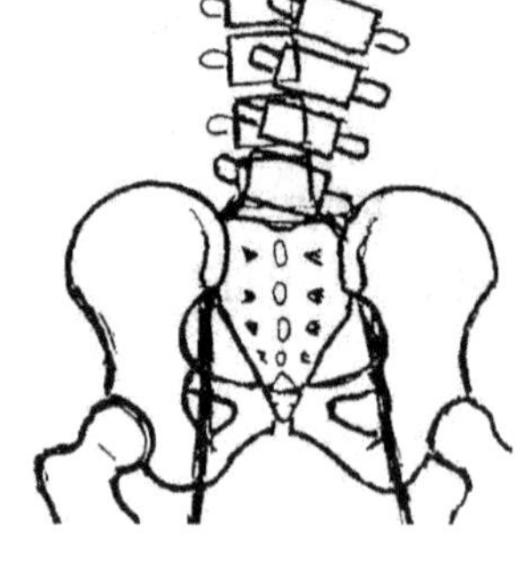

If certain that the Anteriority is a cause of the pain, place both hands on the patient's pelvis whilst still in the PRONE position. Ask the patient to try to raise the buttocks while you resist his efforts for about five seconds at a time. At the end of each time a slight P to A thrust is given. Three times is sufficient.

DO NOT ATTEMPT THIS IF THE PATIENT IS IN GREAT PAIN.

It is often found that patients with low back pain exhibiting spondylolisthesis on X-Ray, test positive for a CAT II and respond well to the SUPINE BLOCKING.

SACRAL TIPPAGE

Where there is localized backache with or without either unilateral or bilateral sciatica there will be pain lateral to the LIGAMENTUM NUCHAE.

The side of pain would indicate the SACRAL INFERIORITY.

This would require MANUAL CORRECTION.

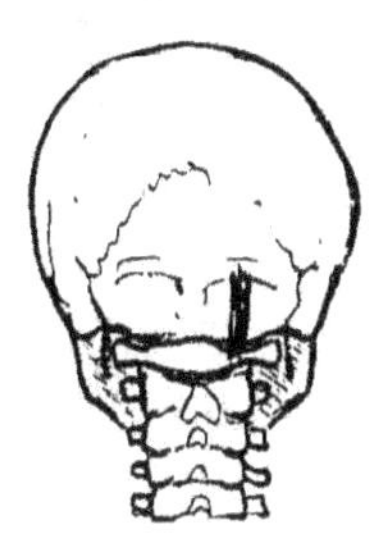

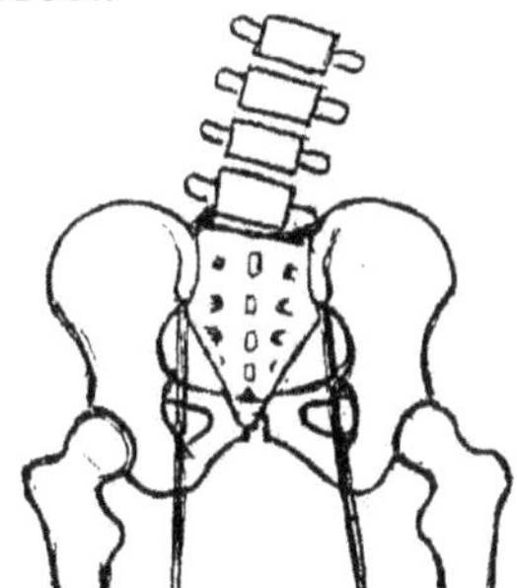

THE PSOAS

The Psoas is often involved with a disc problem, but it can also be the cause of the SCIATICA as can the PIRIFORMIS.

During the examination you checked the PSOAS by the ARMS TEST or by the AK muscle test and found them uneven.

The patient is often pulled forward and is unable to raise the leg.

There is also pain on sitting or walking.

PAIN PATTERNS

With LUMBAR TIPPAGE pain will be found on both of the STYLOIDS or both of the AXIS TRANSVERSES or both of the C3 TRANSVERSES.

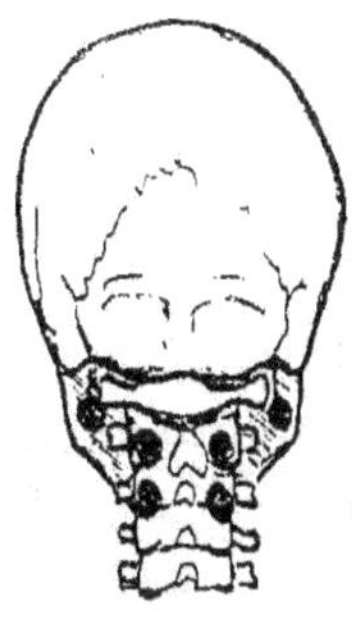

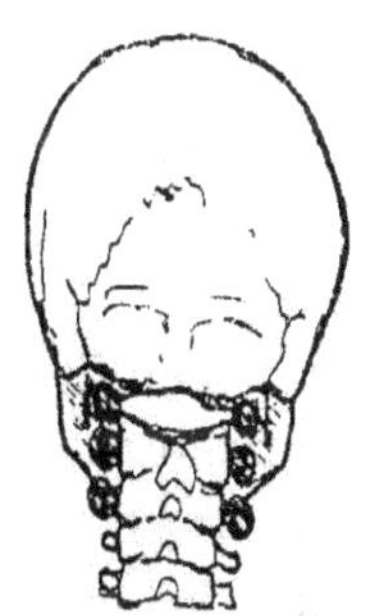

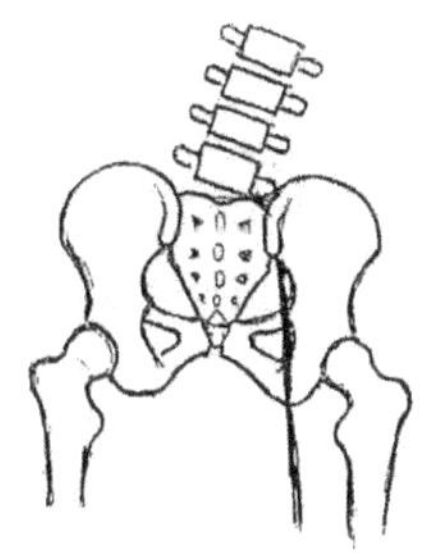

With LUMBAR ROTATION pain will be found on both of the ATLAS, AXIS or C3 TRANSVERSES.

The PSOAS CORRECTION has been described fully under CAT I. It can be done following the BLOCKING and is best done on the second or third visit.

PIRIFORMIS

The PIRIFORMIS can sometimes become stretched and sag, causing pressure on the SCIATIC NERVE by a pincer- type action. This is fairly common, so be aware of it.

The patient feels a scatter type pain in the SACRO-LUMBAR AREA, THE HIP JOINT, GLUTEALS AND UPPER LEG.

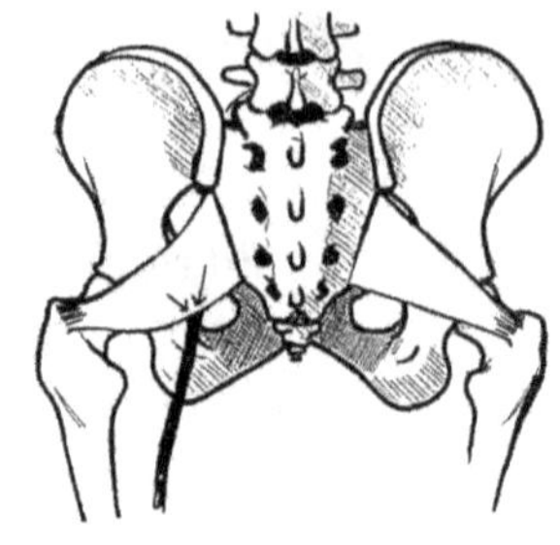

Elongated PIRIFORMIS putting pressure on the Sciatic Nerve

The Posture is normal but pain is aggravated by standing and body movements. If the blocking does not relieve the pain, then the best correction is the STEP-OUT-TOE-OUT (SOTO) technique.

THE STEP-OUT-TOE-OUT TECHNIQUE (SOTO)

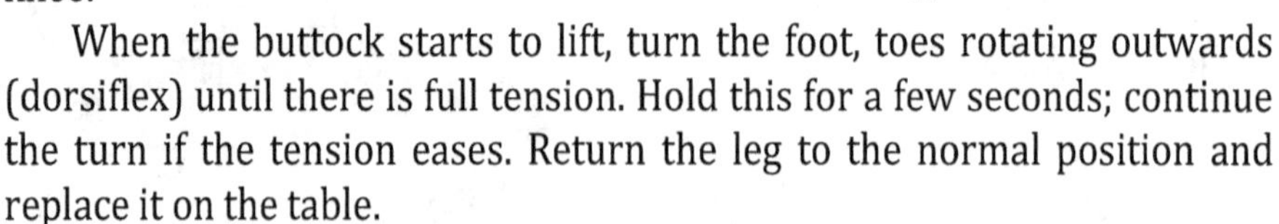

If the second or third attempt reduces the pain, it means that the Piriformis is involved. Stop the blocking now. Do nothing else today.

While the patient is on the blocks for the CAT III placement, grasp the leg on the SCIATICA SIDE by the knee and the foot.

Bring the leg laterally, supporting the knee.

When the buttock starts to lift, turn the foot, toes rotating outwards (dorsiflex) until there is full tension. Hold this for a few seconds; continue the turn if the tension eases. Return the leg to the normal position and replace it on the table.

Repeat this maneuver a few times during the blocking. If there is pain on the first attempt do not be alarmed, this is probably a good sign and the second SOTO will be easier.

If the second or third attempt reduces the pain, it means that the Piriformis *is* involved. Stop the Blocking, and do nothing else today.

OTHER CAUSES OF SCIATICA

If two or three attempts at the SOTO do not relieve the pain or make it worse check for other causes, including:

A vasomotor subluxation: If the SOTO causes pain in the Thoracic spine check for a Vasomotor Subluxation by the Occipital Line method (Covered in CAT I) and adjust.

Extremities: The Tarsals or Fibula could be involved.

Respiratory fixation: Here's where the Cough test could help, where applicable, to find a SB + or - fault. If pain permits, do the Cough test and change the blocks accordingly. Flex the knee and pump the foot, dorsi-flexing the toes, three times then complete the SB+ or SB –.

Disc Fragmentation: A disc fragment may be catching the nerve. If blocking and SOTO do not shift it, refer for surgery, do not try to adjust it.

If there was NO INCREASE and NO DECREASE in the pain level, look for:

- A Positive Calf Sign.
- Flaccid Leg.
- Atrophy of the leg muscles.
- Numbness or circulatory failure.

THESE COULD BE SIGNS OF A NUCLEUS PULPOSUS HERNIATION WITH POSSIBLE CALCIFICATION. SURGERY WOULD BE INDICATED.

THE ILEOFEMORAL LIGAMENT

A very useful technique for both CAT I and Cat III is the ILEOFEMORAL LIGAMENT ADJUSTMENT. If there is severe Sciatica, take a moment whilst measuring the leg lengths and medially rotate the feet, (toes move medially). If there is restriction in the medial rotation of one of the feet there will be some restriction of motion in the ACETABULUM. There may be pathology so proceed with caution.

Usually there is restriction on the SCIATIC SIDE. If after three attempts with the SOTO there is still restriction in the Acetabular region then the **ILEOFEMORAL LIGAMENT ADJUSTMENT** may do the trick.

PALPATE AROUND THE GREATER TROCHANTER FOR PAINFUL AREAS.

These pain points should be released with thumb pressure and movement, with a goading motion.

Once the pain points have been cleared, make a DOUBLE THUMB CONTACT over the TUBERCLE OF THE GREATER TROCHANTER.

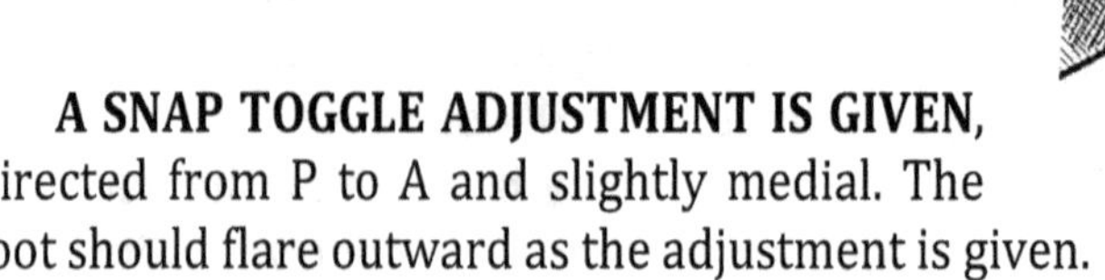

A SNAP TOGGLE ADJUSTMENT IS GIVEN, directed from P to A and slightly medial. The foot should flare outward as the adjustment is given.

SACRAL BASE PLUS MINUS

The Sacral Base or SB + or SB – is covered fully in the CAT I section. The block placement as it relates to the CAT III patient is described here.

Once the blocking time has passed, do the Cough Test (refer to CAT I procedures) only if the patient's condition is relatively stable and a cough will NOT cause pain. A painful cough will not provide any useful information and will only aggravate the patient's condition.

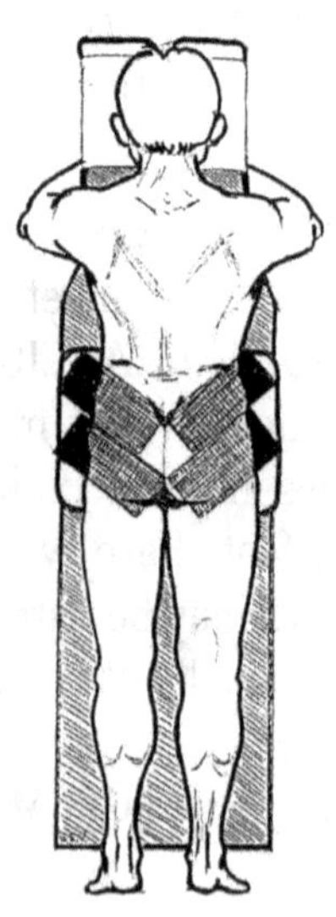

The Cough Test will tell you whether to place the blocks as an SB + or an SB –.

SB +

For the SB + placement remove the inferior (Pedal/Caudal) block and move it superior (Cephalic) to mirror the upper block on the opposite side..

SB -

The SB – placement is of course the reverse. Remove the superior (Cephalic) block and move it inferior to mirror the inferior (Pedal/Caudal) block on the opposite side.

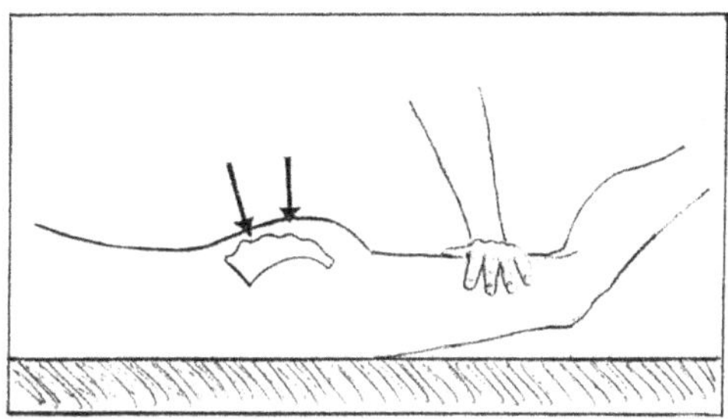

BALANCING THE SACRUM

With the patient prone ask him to raise one straight leg, and test for strength; then test the other. If there is a weakness apply pressure to the superior sacral notch on that side and test for strength again. If there is no improvement apply the pressure to the inferior notch and test again. If either causes the strength to improve then use an activator or your thumb to thrust on that notch.

ONCE THE PATIENT HAS RETURNED TO A PAIN-FREE CONDITION AND SHOWS NO FURTHER SIGN OF CAT III INVOLVEMENT, PROCEED AS WITH A CAT I TO RESTORE THE PATIENT TO A HEALTHY PHYSIOLOGICAL CAT I STATE.

11

CATEGORY I

Welcome to what at first glance appears to be a very simple blocking approach, but what is in fact as near to a holistic technique as one can find within Chiropractic.

The **PATHOLOGICAL CAT I** is the breakdown of the respiratory mechanism in the pelvis. Either there is a Sacro-iliac subluxation (The **DOLLAR** sign) or an llio-sacral subluxation (the **CREST** sign); these will be explained later. Either of these subluxations causes a jamming of the essential motion at the **BOOT** Synovial articulation of the Sacro-iliac.

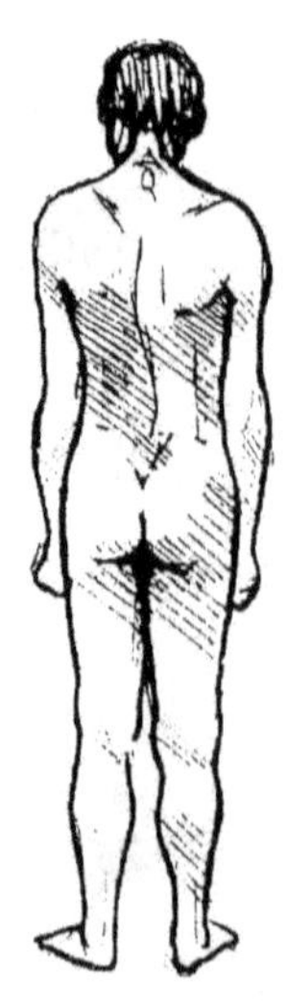

When this **Synovial diarthrodial articulation** is jammed, the respiratory motion is lost in the pelvis that can create a reciprocal distortion in the Cranium, and the body desperately tries to compensate for the loss of the essential CSF pump action.

Remember the CSF pump mechanism extends from the Ventricles of the brain to the Dura Mater in the Cranium and the Spinal cord to the Sacrum. If one part is distorted the whole system becomes affected, so the Chiropractor must think in terms of the entire system.

The Blocking helps the patient to correct this fault during the respiratory cycle. It is the breathing during the blocking that actually starts the correction. The whole CAT I procedure should be used to find and correct the various types of vertebral subluxation, the Cranial faults as well as the soft tissue reflexes.

To fully understand CAT I requires a dedication justly rewarded. The placement of the blocks is but the beginning of a system of analysis and treatment involving the entire spine and the bones of the cranium. It also involves the entire nervous system and the wellbeing of the patient.

The patient exhibiting a PATHOLOGICAL CAT I problem is a sick person. He may be just a little off-colour or even symptom-free, but if he has been a CAT I for a long time he could be very sick and have active pathology at work in the body.

A HEALTHY CAT I IS THE AIM OF THE CHIROPRACTOR.

It is essential to return a CAT II or CAT III to the CAT I state and then clear out any distortions within CAT I, so that the patient is discharged as a healthy PHYSIOLOGICAL CATEGORY l.

EXAMINATION FINDINGS

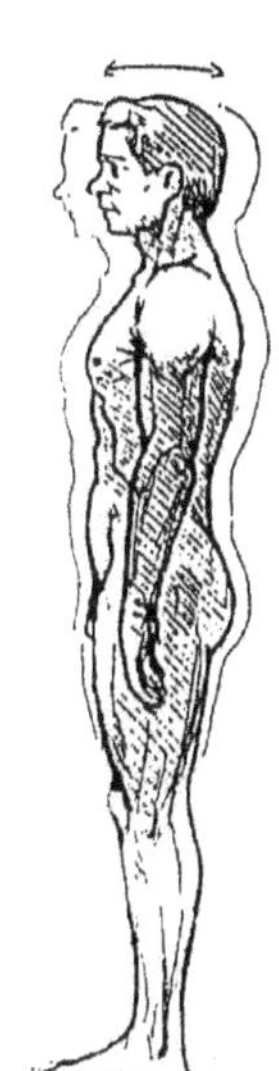

On examination there is an AP sway whilst standing with eyes closed.

The pelvis does not sway and appears intact.

The patient stands erect but there may be some scoliosis.

Both rib heads are mobile to touch and possibly sore when the patient hyper-flexes and hyper-extends the neck.

The head may be held as if it is heavy.

The **MIND LANGUAGE TEST** is positive on the first position, when the PSS is contacted.

There is a short leg in the prone position and there is heel tension on one side, usually the same side as the short leg but not always.

CATEGORY I

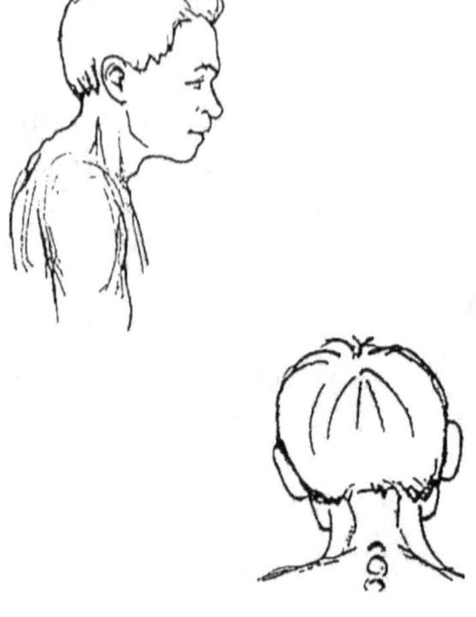

The case history may have ranged from Low Back Pain, Sciatica, or pains in any part of the spine. Questioning may have revealed internal disorders, headaches, disturbed sleep or just about any form of discomfort or dis-ease.

Remember this is a sick or potentially sick patient.

12

CATEGORY I CORRECTION

CAT I CORRECTION

The **PELVIC BOARD** should be in place beneath the pelvis and the **STERNAL ROLL** should be positioned so that it lies directly beneath the patient's chest.

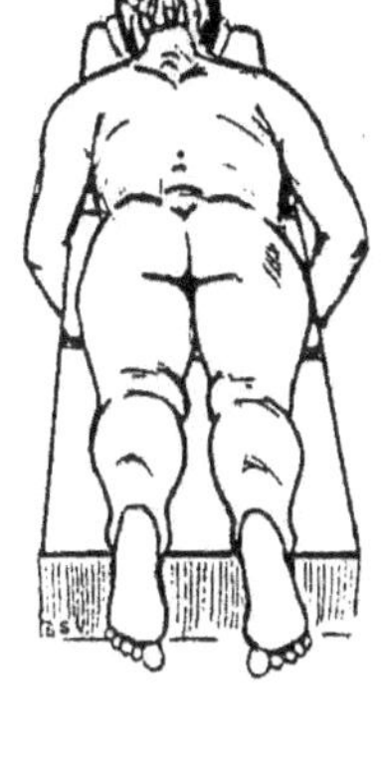

Place the patient PRONE. Make sure that the Pelvic Board is positioned so that the Pelvis is centered on it.

Check that the Sternal Roll is also Centered; make sure it does not put pressure on the trachea.

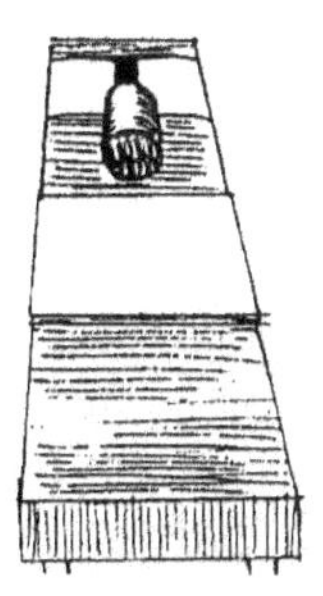

Make sure that the patient is lying straight and relaxed; be patient especially if this is the first visit.

Explain what you are doing and ask the patient to become involved. A patient cannot relax if he is waiting for the unexpected.

LEG LENGTH AND HEEL TENSION

Grasp both ankles, fingers below and thumbs across the Achilles tendon just superior to its attachment to the Calcaneous.

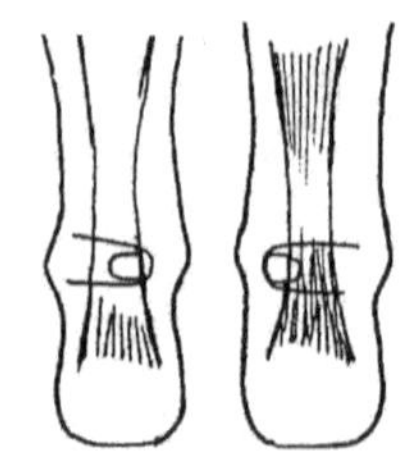

Exert a firm but gentle pull equally on both legs. Gaze along the body to ensure that the patient is straight, head pointed down and shoulders relaxed. Release the pull on the legs but with hands still in place. Feel for a tense Achilles tendon, which can often be seen before palpation.

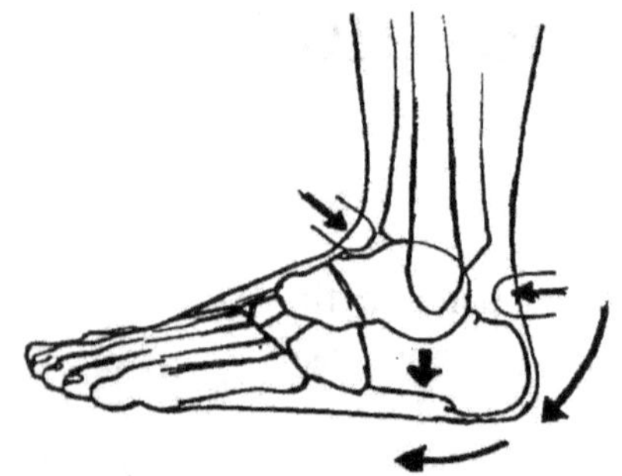

One side will be tense in a CAT I. Record this as the **Heel Tension** (HT) side.

Bend the knees, push the heels towards the buttocks and then bring the legs to the vertical. Flex the feet and feel for more resistance on one side.

CATEGORY I BLOCKING

THE SHORT LEG BLOCK is placed beneath the ACETABULUM pointing towards the opposite ASIS.

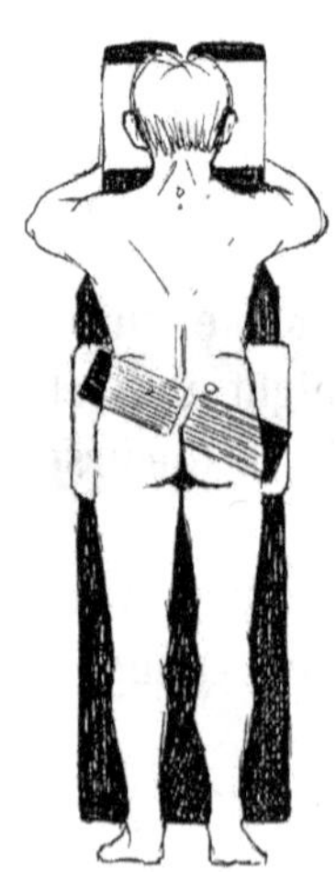

THE LONG LEG BLOCK is placed beneath the ASIS pointing towards the end of the SHORT LEG BLOCK.

HEEL TENSION TECHNIQUE

Grasp the **HEEL TENSION LEG** with a contact the same as when you were measuring for HEEL TENSION. Ask the patient to hold the top of the table whilst pulling the HEEL TENSION LEG, flexing the foot slightly as you do it. Then release and get the patient to relax.

The short leg should equalize within seconds. If it does not, remove the blocks and re-assess leg lengths. If necessary, have the patient walk around for a while before re-measuring.

Once satisfied that the blocking is correct, instruct the patient to relax and breathe normally.

RIGHT SHORT LEG

ONCE THE HEEL TENSION HAS EASED AND THE LEGS HAVE EQUALIZED OR CHANGED (SOMETIMES THE SHORT WILL APPEAR LONG DURING THE BLOCKING) IT IS TIME TO TEST AND TREAT THE CRESTS AND DOLLARS.

THE CREST SIGN

The CRESTS are the Iliac Crests where the Quadratus Lumborum muscles attach. The **CREST SIGNS** indicate that there is a MUSCULO-SKELETAL problem. The pelvic distortion is an ILIO-SACRAL subluxation. This CREST SIGN also indicates that if a Cranial adjustment is required it will be to the TEMPORAL BONES.

Get used to looking for the CRESTS; they are highly significant. There are two things to look for in the CRESTS:

Pain over the ILIAC CRESTS: Palpate by THUMB PRESSURE along the length of both ILIAC CRESTS, from lateral to medial (the Davis Stretch Sign) and ask the patient which is more painful. **The side OPPOSITE THE PAINFUL SIDE is the MAJOR CREST SIDE. The side of PAIN is the side for treatment.**

Tension along the QUADRATUS LUMBORUM MUSCLES: Contact the Medial borders of the Lumbar musculature with four fingers on either side. PULL LATERALLY and feel for the HIGH or TENSE SIDE (The Davis Contractile Sign). **The TENSE SIDE is the MAJOR. The Flaccid side is the TREATMENT SIDE.**

If there is either PAIN or TENSION in the CRESTS then they require some treatment at this stage of the Blocking.

If the PAINFUL SIDE is also the FLACCID SIDE, place your thumb on the LATERAL margin of the Quadratus Lumborum and press medially towards the 4th Lumbar spinous. Work the thumb with a goading pressure for thirty seconds.

If the PAINFUL SIDE is the TENSE SIDE then hold the thumb as before but exert a constant pressure without goading for thirty seconds.

NOW GO TO THE DOLLAR SIGNS

THE DOLLAR SIGN

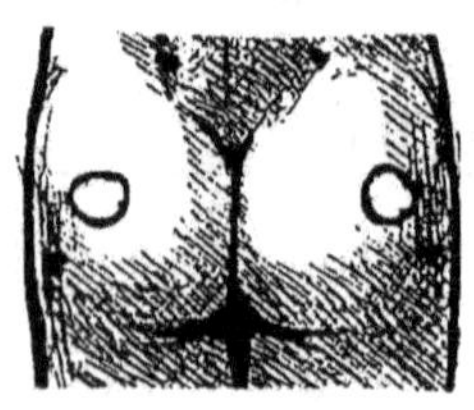

THE DOLLAR SIGN is named, not for its shape but because of its size. It is about the size of a US SILVER DOLLAR COIN.

The Dollar **Sign indicates a SACRO-ILIAC problem and a NEUROLOGICAL disturbance**. The Sacral part of the Boot mechanism is jammed and the essential nodding motion impaired. Where Cranial bones are involved it will be the CENTRAL BONES OF THE SKULL.

The area to examine is in each buttock, at the point where the fibers of the Gluteal muscles and the Piriformis cross. Imagine a line stretching from the PSIS to the GREATER TROCHANTER; two thirds of the way along this line is an area about the size of a silver dollar. This is the Dollar sign. Once again we are looking for two things: PAIN and TENSION.

LOOKING FOR PAIN

THE PRESSURE TECHNIQUE is a deep pressure with the thumb in both Dollar Signs. Palpate for the most painful side.

LOOKING FOR TENSION

The TAP TECHNIQUE is a performed by tapping the DOLLAR with the forefinger, looking for either a firmness or dullness. Do it as if you were tapping a partition looking for the place to put a nail. **The FIRM side is the MAJOR. The Dull or Flabby side is the side needing treatment.**

USUALY THE PAINFUL SIDE IS ALSO THE FLABBY SIDE.

CATEGORY I CORRECTION

TREATING THE PAINFUL DOLLAR SIDE

Press the index finger into the PAINFUL dollar. Make a circular motion, with as much pressure as the patient can stand until the pain eases. There will always be some pain in the dollar area, so don't go for perfection.

LET THE PATIENT REMAIN ON THE BLOCKS FOR 4 TO 5 MINUTES.

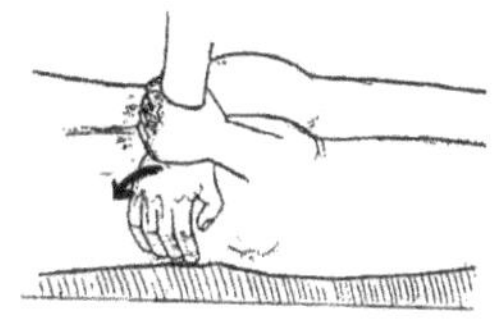

The thrust is a ROLL ACTION over the CREST with the direction being towards the head.

THIS ADJUSTMENT WOULD ALWAYS BE MADE ON THE SIDE OF THE SHORT LEG (LOWER BLOCK).

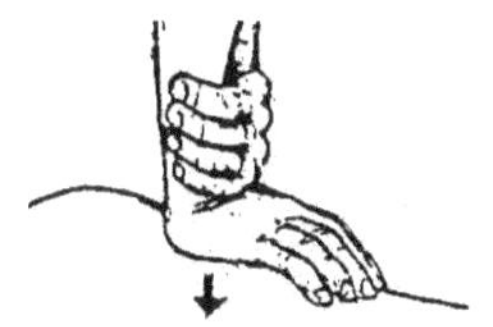

Also a flat hand contact onto the ISCHIUM with a thrust directly down onto the ISHIUM.

ADJUST THE MAJOR SIDE FIRST.

The Blocks will let you know which adjustment to make. Use your common sense; you cannot thrust into a block. Therefore, if the MAJOR SIDE is on the SHORT LEG SIDE (LOW BLOCK SIDE) the CREST Adjustment would be indicated FIRST. Adjust the CREST, and then adjust the ISCHIUM.

Once the Crests and Dollars have been checked and treated leave the patient to relax on the Blocks for four or five minutes, perhaps see another patient or just relax as well.

When you return to the patient, recheck the Crests and Dollars. At this stage the attempt is to determine which is more involved. Remember **the CRESTS indicate that the Iliac has subluxated on the Sacrum (Ilio-sacral) and the DOLLARS indicate that the Sacrum is subluxated between the Ilia (Sacro-iliac).**

Some experience will be required to make this decision but start looking right now.

ONCE YOU HAVE DECIDED WHICH NEEDS TO BE ADJUSTED MAKE THE ADJUSTMENT. IT IS EITHER THE DOLLAR OR THE CREST NOT BOTH.

THE CREST ADJUSTMENT

There are TWO PARTS OF THE ADJUSTMENT.

A flat hand contact is made along the length of the Crest. The little finger contacts the Crest itself with the remainder of the hand contacting the Ilium.

Also a flat hand contact onto the ISCHIUM. The thrust is directly down onto the ISCHIUM.

THE COUGH TEST

This is the **VASOMOTOR TECHNIQUE** to determine whether the SACRAL BASE is caught in EXTENSION, i.e. at the point of maximum EXHALATION (SB+), OR FLEXION at the point of maximum INHALATION (SB –).

When the Sacral base is at an angle of more than 34º from the horizontal it is more likely to find an SB +. When less than 30º an SB – is more likely. BUT SB problems are MEMBRANE problems and not FACET problems, so DO NOT rely on X-ray measurement of Sacral Base angle (Ferguson's angle).

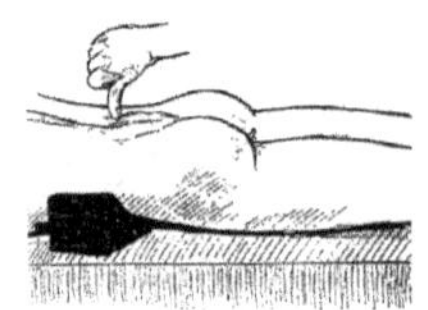

With the patient still on the Blocks, point a locked thumb directly downward onto the spinous of L5, the contact is just enough to make bone contact. Have the patient grasp the head of the table, take a deep breath and pull strongly with the arms. Ask the patient to COUGH. Watch your thumb to see whether it is pushed:

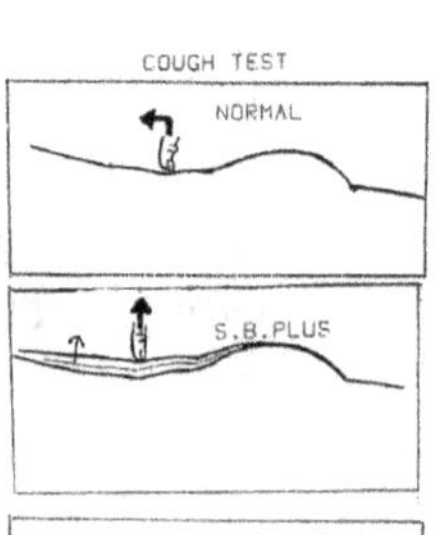

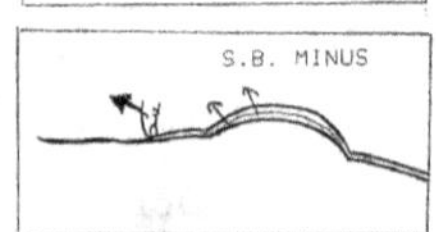

Straight up and then towards the head. NORMAL.

Straight up. The Lumbar vertebrae seem to move together.

SB + The Sacrum is locked in EXTENSION at the limit of EXHALATION.

SB - The Sacrum is locked in FLEXION, at the limit of INHALATION.

CHANGING THE BLOCKS

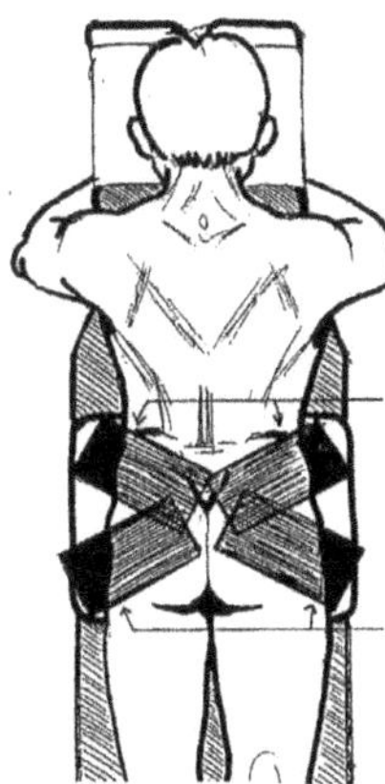

SB + The LOWER BLOCK is moved to mirror the higher block.
BOTH BLOCKS ARE IN THE **HIGHER POSITION.**

SB - The HIGHER BLOCK is moved to mirror the LOWER BLOCK.
BOTH BLOCKS ARE IN THE **LOWER POSITION**.

To assist in the SB adjustment, place your hand onto the Sacrum and ask the patient to breathe deeply but regularly. As you feel the rhythm of the breathing allow your hand to follow the movement of the Sacrum and assist:

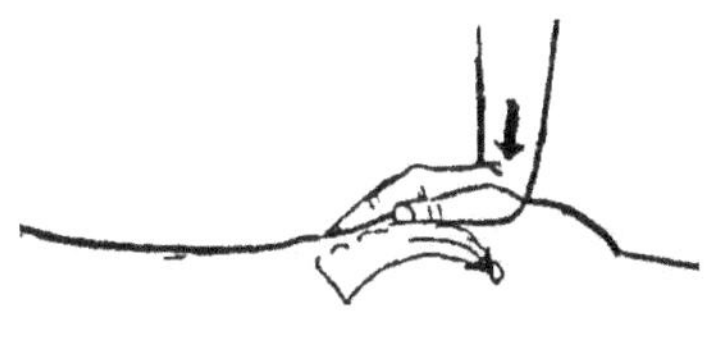

SB + on **INSPIRATION** with the pressure at the apex of the Sacrum. Remember the SB + is stuck in Extension and so needs help into **Flexion**.

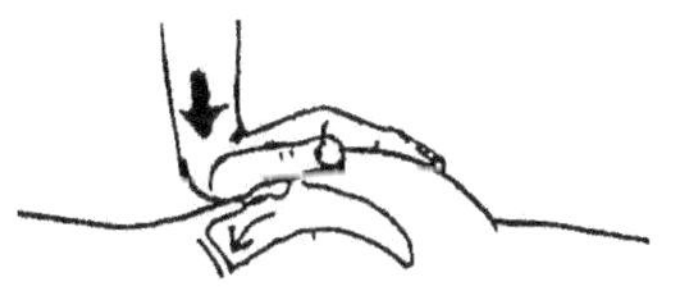

SB - on **EXPIRATION** with the pressure at the base of the Sacrum. The SB - is stuck in Flexion and so needs help into **Extension**.

LOOKING FOR THE VASOMOTOR SUBLUXATION

After a few respiratory cycles, ask the patient to reach up and grasp the head of the table, inhale and pull to create traction along the spine. Your hand is still on the Sacrum for the SB adjustment.

If there is an **SB +** then the pressure is placed on the **Apex** of the Sacrum.

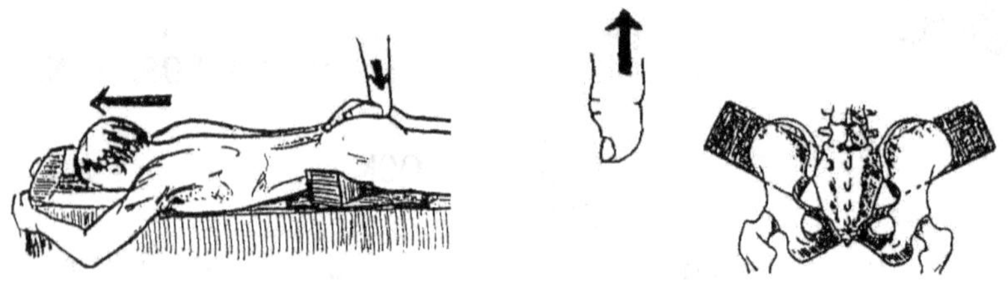

If there is an **SB –** then the pressure is placed on the **Base** of the Sacrum.

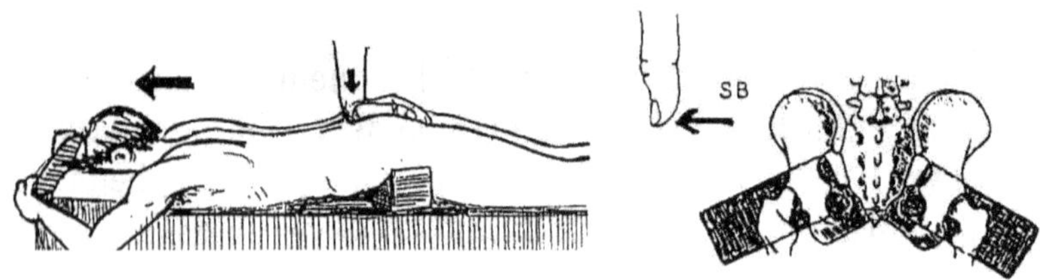

HOLD THE PRESSURE FOR FOUR SECONDS.

Look for BLANCHING of the skin over the spine. There may be just one or several. The blanching should cross the vertebra. If it is centered over the spinous process then the adjustment will be made to the spinous. If the Blanching is centered over the Transverse Process then the adjustment will be to the Transverse.

IF MORE THAN ONE BLANCHED VERTEBRA, ADJUST THE MOST SUPERIOR FIRST; THEN RECHECK FOR BLANCHING BEFORE ADJUSTING THE NEXT.

THE BLANCHED VERTEBRAE are in VASOMOTOR SUBLUXATION.

This is part of the fascinating Visceral approach to Chiropractic, which warrants a book of its own. Dr. Major de Jarnette's book *CMRT* is a good start for future study.

The blanched vertebrae usually agree with those found by the OCCIPITAL LINE technique. If after adjusting the Vasomotors the Occipital line fibers have not eased then the OCCIPITAL LINE TECHNIQUE is needed.

The OCCIPITAL LINE TECHNIQUE is introduced at the end of this Chapter as it is a most important tool for the Chiropractor.

THE VASOMOTOR ADJUSTMENT

The STERNAL ROLL should be in place; this is when it comes into its own. The only exception for the Sternal Roll is for a very KYPHOTIC thoracic spine.

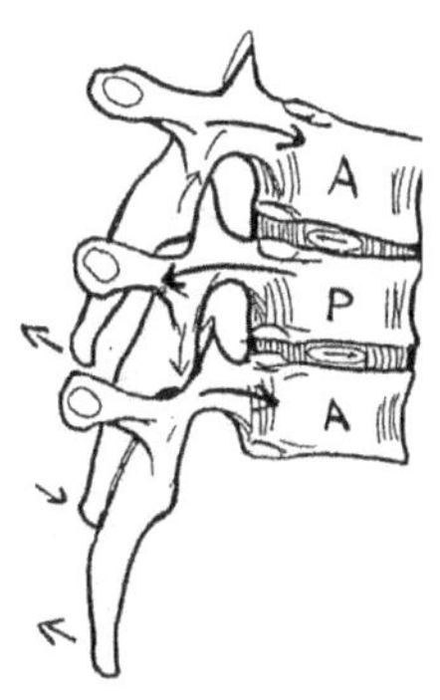

When you locate a BLANCHED vertebra, palpate it and those adjacent. If the Blanching was centered over the spinous, then a painful spinous will be found, usually where there is a depression (POTTENGER'S SAUCER). When the Blanching is centered over the transverse, then a painful and prominent transverse will be found.

As Dr. Pottenger described the saucer it was named after him when he noted that such a saucer was always associated with visceral disease.

The depression is a combination of Anterior and Posterior vertebrae. The vertebrae above and below the most dipped are Anterior in relation to the one in the middle. The spinous process that palpates as being anterior belongs to a vertebra that is in fact posterior. As the body moves to the posterior the spinous must be forced inferior and anterior and so is closer to the spinous of the vertebra below.

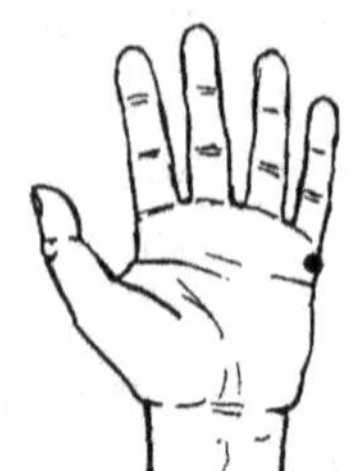

THE CONTACT is a knife-edge nail point #1.

THE THRUST will be a lifting scoop with the contact tucked well under the spinous and delivered in the following manner:

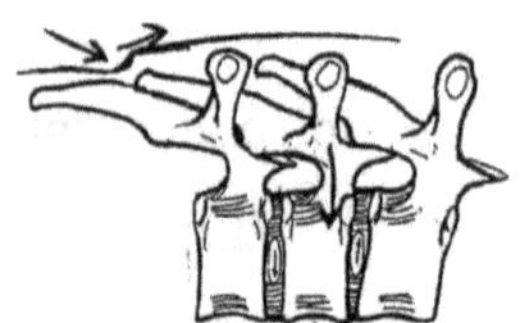

SB + FULL INSPIRATION as the patient starts to **EXHALE.** The Blocks are still in the **higher position**.

SB - FULL EXPIRATION as the patient starts to **INHALE**. The Blocks are still in the **lower position**.

After the adjustment **RECHECK FOR BLANCHING**. The most superior should be adjusted first. Then recheck to see if that adjustment also cleared out the others; if not then adjust the next blanched vertebra down. Continue to check and adjust until all blanched vertebrae are cleared.

This is not a heavy adjustment. When done correctly with the right respiratory cycle, there is often a spontaneous unlocking of the subluxation, just with the contact pressure alone and no thrust is required.

Where the thrust is required, the drive is just enough to do the unlocking. If the curve of the Thoracic spine is normal or flattened then the direction is superior, sliding up towards the head. If there is an exaggerated kyphosis, the line of drive will be almost directly A to P.

A flattened, lordotic spine is more likely to be associated with the SB– whilst the rounded, kyphotic spine with SB +.

13

THE OCCIPITAL LINE TECHNIQUE

The Vasomotor subluxations, found during the Blocking procedure, will often coincide with the Occipital Line Indicators. A careful study of the Occipital Lines however can lead to a more thorough understanding of the patient's health problems, as well as open doors to further procedures to help restore him to health.

Herein is a mere introduction to the OCCIPITAL LINES and the adjustive procedures that accompany them. This is an area that warrants considerable study and leads into a reflex approach to visceral problems.

Once familiar with the basic SOT approach, continue study of Dr. De Jarnette's *CMRT and Cranial work.*

FINDING THE LINES

The best time to make this examination is whilst the patient is lying prone on the blocks. The examiner sits at the head of the table facing the top of the patient's head.

There are seven fibers, equally placed between the medial aspcct of the mastoid and the lateral Nuchal borders on each side, level with the upper third of the ear.

These fibers run vertically starting as part of the musculature and ending in the Aponeurosis.

The fibers are bisected by two imaginary lines to give us the LINE ONE, LINE TWO and LINE THREE.

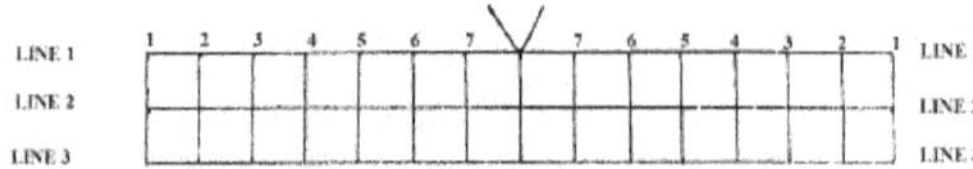

Place the index finger immediately medial to the Occipito-mastoid suture at the level of line one (the Mastoid Vee), then place the second finger immediately below it to exert a slight downward skin tension. Now use the index finger to palpate for the first fiber.

The skin tension should allow for going on to find the second fiber, and when found bring the second finger across to renew the skin tension at the second fiber. Remember both hands are working together palpating from both mastoids.

These fibers are distinguishable and you should be able to locate each one. Move carefully, the fibers are quite close to each other and require careful palpation to identify. Look for a fiber that is tighter than the rest. When you find a tight fiber, slide your finger down to the next level to see if there is any nodulation.

LINE ONE

Line one is the uppermost of the three lines and the fibers are felt as thin not easily defined separate strands within the Aponeurosis.

The one you are looking for is slightly raised and feels tense. The patient will usually feel pain when you find it. If the musculature below the Line One is not nodulated then you have a LINE ONE FIBRE.

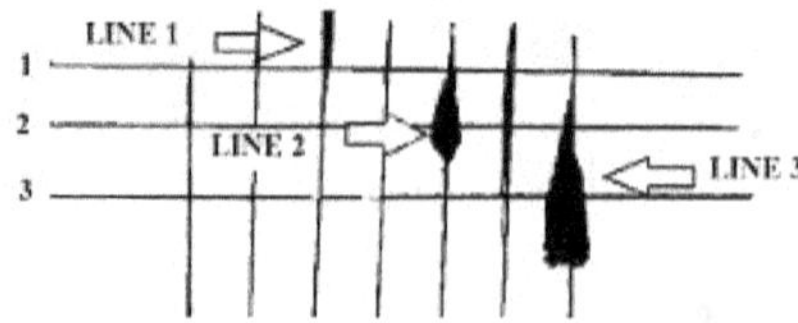

There are various factors that you must decide when finding a painful fiber or fibers:

Which fiber? Counting is from Lateral to Medial, seven on either side.

Which Line? One Two or Three.

Which side, Left or Right?

Are there one, or more fibers involved?

The LINE ONE fiber signals a CNS flow and Dural Torque problem probably associated with one of the Categories and is usually resolved by the Category technique.

If it is not resolved then an adjustment to lift the spinous of the offending vertebra is given. See the LINE ONE Adjustment Technique diagram.

LINE TWO

Once a taut and tender fiber on line one is found with the palpating finger, slide the finger down a little to see if there is a thickened nodule at the second horizontal level which is LINE TWO.

When line two is involved, what was a relatively minor or acute problem has become a more serious or chronic problem in which visceral involvement has begun. Prompt treatment can reverse the process. See the LINE TWO Adjustment Technique diagram.

LINE THREE

If instead of the nodule in line two, a thickened muscle that extends down to the third level is found, it is a more serious problem in which a pathological process could be involved.

Warning bells should ring and a thorough examination of the patient is necessary, with particular attention being paid to the organ indicated by the LINE THREE FIBRE. See the LINE THREE Adjustment Technique diagram.

IDENTIFYING RELATED VERTEBRAE AND VISCERA

The seven fibers relate to the seven cervical vertebrae, which in turn relate to thoracic and lumbar vertebrae. Remember that the relationships are not absolute and careful palpation of the indicated vertebra and the ones above and below is necessary to determine the one to adjust if required.

It is also important to remember that there is variation between different authorities regarding which segment relates to which organ. There is of course a complex circuitry in the Autonomic Nervous System, so that several segmental levels are involved with every organ.

SEE APPENDIX D

OCCIPITAL	1	2	3	4	5	6	7
CERVICAL	1	2	3	4	5	6	7
DORSAL	1, 2,10	3, 11, 12	4-5	6	7	8	9
LUMBAR			1	2	3	4	5

LINE ONE ADJUSTING TECHNIQUE

Once you have identified a LINE ONE FIBRE, refer to the chart and test each of the thoracic and lumbar vertebrae that relate to that fiber. As an example of this, say you have found a taut number four fiber on line one. The thoracic vertebra would be the sixth (T6) and the lumbar vertebra would be the second (L2).

For a NORMAL or FLATTENED thoracic curve a STERNAL ROLL is placed under the patient. The subluxation is a posteriority of the body of the vertebra with the spinous being forced inferior and anterior against the spinous of the vertebra below.

Testing for the major is done by locating the relative spinous and forcing it further into subluxation, inferior and anterior. This will elicit pain and a burning sensation, you must decide which of the vertebrae tested caused more discomfort. Muscle testing can also be used here.

The Major spinous is then contacted with the thumb just inferior to the tip of the spinous, pointing directly up the spine towards the head, the remainder of the hand lies on the back. The other hand locates the relative cervical vertebra with finger and thumb and holds lightly.

With the previous example of the fourth fiber, the thumb will be contacting either the sixth thoracic or the second lumbar and the other hand will be holding the fourth cervical vertebra.

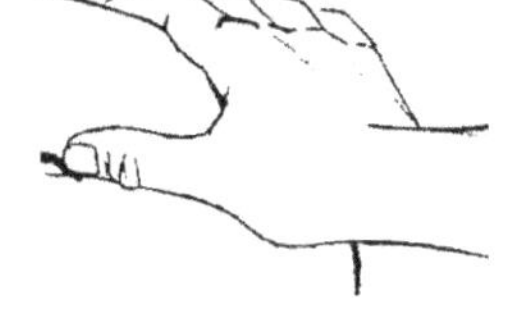

As the patient inhales the thumb moves the spinous tip headwards. As the patient exhales the pressure is released. Continue this rhythm until you feel a moisture at the cervical contact.

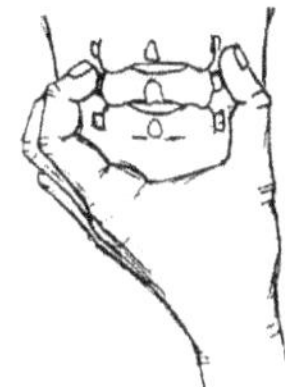

The movement of the thumb can be done by anchoring the hand on the patient's back, then bend and straighten the thumb. You are not trying to make a correction but merely a pumping motion.

Once the moisture is felt, release the cervical hand make a nail point #1 contact on the spinous, support it with the other hand and ask the patient to inhale once more and exhale completely. The correction is the same as for the

SACRAL BASE TECHNIQUE, the thrust is headward as you attempt to scoop the spinous tip away from the one below and drive it superior. The body will then be forced to move anterior and inferior.

THE KYPHOTIC SPINE does not require the sternal roll and the subluxation is the opposite to that of the normal or flattened spine. The movement of the body is anterior, thus forcing the spinous posterior and superior. The PUMP is done during exhalation with the direction of force being anterior and inferior. The adjustment is also anterior and inferior.

Very often the LINE ONE fiber subluxation coincides with the SB subluxation and was taken care of by the SB technique.

LINE TWO ADJUSTING TECHNIQUE

OCCIPITAL	1	2	3	4	5	6	7
DORSAL	1, 2, 9, 10	3, 11, 12	4, 5	6	7	8	9
LUMBAR			1	2	(3)	4	(5)
			↕	↕		↕	
SACRAL			1	2		4	

When you locate a line two nodule look to the chart and examine the thoracic and lumbar vertebrae indicated and find the major.

The LINE TWO subluxation is a rotation with one high usually painful transverse. Palpate for the most prominent transverse.

The STERNAL ROLL is used for all patients except for those with a dorsal kyphosis.

Remember this is a patient with some pathological changes; they may not be diagnosable changes at this point, so are most responsive to the line two technique followed by CMRT.

For your own comfort it is best to sit at the patient's side whilst doing this technique.

Contact the LINE TWO FIBRE with the index finger of one hand whilst the other hand contacts the HIGH TRANSVERSE of the major vertebra. This contact is also with the index finger.

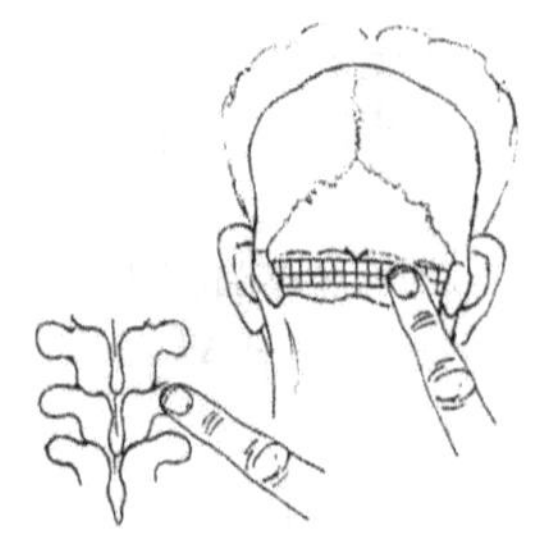

The TRANSVERSE HAND maintains contact whilst the OCCIPITAL HAND vigorously massages the line two fiber. This will be quite painful but the pain will decrease after a while.

Continue with the line two until the finger contacting the vertebra feels warm and moist.

Then adjust the vertebra to take out the rotation.

OCCIPITAL	1	2	3	4	5	6	7
DORSAL	1, 2, 9, 10	3, 11, 12	4, 5	6	7	8	9
LUMBAR			1	2	(3)	4	(5)
			↕	↕		↕	
SACRAL			1	2		4	

Note the Lumbar/Sacral lines on the chart. Where there is an arrow joining a lumbar vertebra with a Sacral segment, then pressure is held at the Sacral level during the line two vibration and then the Lumbar vertebra is adjusted. The Lumbar vertebrae, that have no arrow connecting them to a Sacral segment, are both held and adjusted as were the thoracic vertebrae.

Following the adjustment Chiropractic Manipulative Reflex Technique would help to restore the offending organ to function. This is an involved technique and I suggest you study Dr. De Jarnette's book on the subject.

LINE THREE ADJUSTING TECHNIQUE

In any Line Three problem, the Atlas and Axis should be carefully checked and corrected where indicated.

OCCIPITAL	1	2	3	4	5	6	7
DORSAL	1, 12	2, 11	3, 10	4, 9	7	5, 8	6, 7
LUMBAR	5	4	3	2	1		
CERVICAL	1-2	1-2	1-2	1-2		1-2	1-2

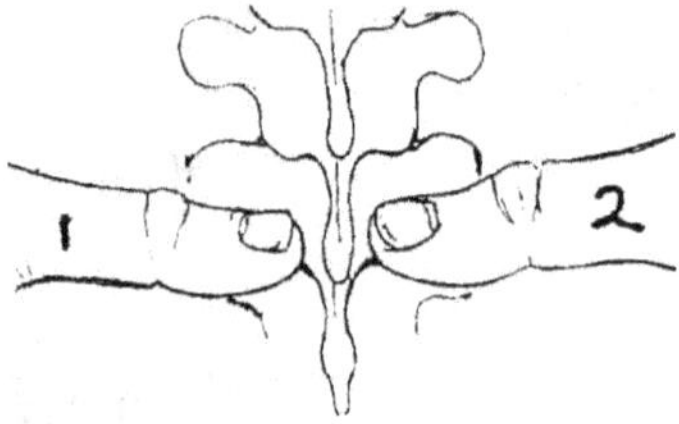

Test the spinous processes of the identified vertebrae. To do this, apply thumb pressure medially from one side and then the other. Note which side is more painful.

Whilst maintaining a steady pressure with the thumb from the side that elicited the greatest pain, contact the transverse of Atlas and then Axis with about half the pressure used below.

If the pain felt at the spinous process being held is reduced by the Atlas or Axis pressure, then the pain was of spinal origin and this technique will help the problem.

Once the pain has subsided, adjust to correct the rotation of the vertebra. Following this, adjust either Atlas or Axis, whichever helped to control the pain.

If the pain at the spinous process does not abate after a reasonable time, then further investigation should be done. Do not attempt to adjust until your are sure there is nothing sinister.

Just as the CAT III problem is an area that requires the full diagnostic consideration, with the necessity of referral, a distinct and realistic possibility.

The **CAT I LINE THREE** demands special attention and referral is recommended where any doubt exists.

14

THE ART OF MUSCLE TESTING

There are believers and skeptics of muscle testing. Some people have taken muscle testing to extreme lengths, which can stretch the limits of anyone's belief system, but here we are using it as part of an assessment for structural changes in the body that need Chiropractic care. Each test result is a pointer to assist in the final diagnosis. Three positions are used for the tests: standing, lying prone and lying supine. The muscle testing is part of the picture and not the whole. Careful history taking and physical examination including, where indicated, X-rays, MRIs and lab tests, are essential for the thorough evaluation of the patient.

One of the most important considerations is the examiner's mindset. It has been shown that the examiner can influence the outcome by projecting his/her preconceived desired outcome. By this I mean that if the examiner has, during the course of the examination so far, decided that the patient has a Category Two problem, the subconscious desire for the muscle test to prove him/her right could result in a false positive test. It is essential that the examiner stays out of the way and allows the tests to show what they may.

It is important to test the muscle or group of muscles, as with the shoulder/arm test used in SOT, prior to challenging the part in question. Three things must happen simultaneously:

The verbal command, HOLD.

Slight pressure exerted on the examining point.

Pressure exerted on the testing arm.

Muscle tests are not a competition between examiner and the patient to see who can overpower the other. In fact, using just two fingers on the testing arm is usually enough to get the desired result. The test is subtle and the amount of power is minimal. The difference between a strong muscle and a weak one is felt immediately. For the strong muscle, there is an instant positive lock in the muscle, whereas the weak one will show a slight hesitance with a mushy feeling. It is unnecessary to go beyond that instant reaction to prove the point. The experienced examiner will feel the response and so will the patient. It is amusing to see the reaction from a muscular bodybuilding type, who is confident that the doctor could do nothing to overpower him; yet, with just two fingers on his wrist and a slight pressure, he has no defense.

All too often people give up on muscle testing because they have no confidence in it. With practice and experience this very simple set of tests can give the examiner valuable information about what problem presents itself on this occasion. By doing the full range of tests on every visit the doctor has a much better idea of what to do today and what not to do today. The latter is just as important as the former. One must never assume that because the patient exhibited signs of, say, a CAT II on the previous visit, that that is what needs to be done again today. Even the most experienced SOT practitioners have had patients who switch from CAT II to CAT III and back again in subsequent visits. Each set of tests takes about 30 seconds; take the time and reap the rewards.

Remember, very important, when doing a test clear your own mind and get yourself out of the way. You are asking the patient's body for information. The answer must come from the patients innate, not you.

The Glass Hand

One of the problems students have when doing the Fossa Test in the CAT II analysis, is in locating the Inguinal Ligament. This is a sensitive area, which can, in the presence of a CAT II problem, be painful as well. Prodding around to find the structures can be a difficult exercise for both the practitioner and the patient. For this reason use what is called the GLASS HAND.

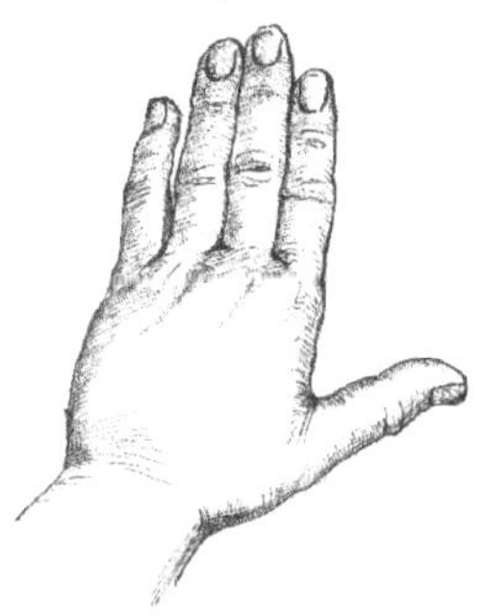

To locate the ASIS without probing into a sensitive area, place the fully extended hand over the area and press gently but firmly until feeling the boney anterior spine of the Ilia. I focus my eye on that part of my hand that lies directly over the ASIS and then while maintaining eye contact on that point, as if looking through a glass hand, move the hand, curling the fingers so that the index finger contacts the point at the ASIS. By sliding the index finger medially, all four fingers should be contacting the lateral half of the Inguinal ligament. Then visualize the pubis, move the hand along the Inguinal Ligament without pressing, until the little finger in on the edge of the pubis; a slight lateral slide will bring the hand in contact with the medial half of the Inguinal Ligament.

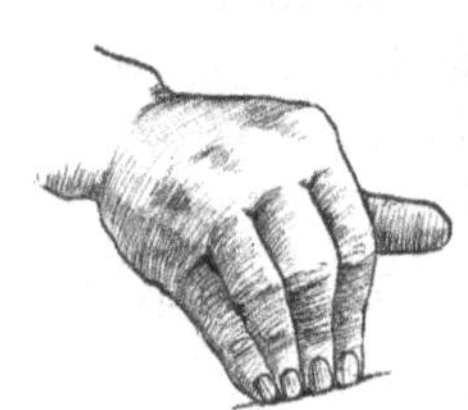

Testing in the prone position

There are a number of muscle tests that are useful while the patient is in the prone position. These are not strictly SOT tests. There are twelve points to test that can give you a wealth of information about the patient lying in front of you. The muscle test is the same, with one arm out to the side, exactly the same as the mind language test standing. Once you have established that the testing arm is strong and there is no shoulder pains etc, then start the test.

Right PSIS, direct pressure towards the table.

Right Ischium, direct pressure towards the table.

Left PSIS, direct pressure towards the table.

Left Ischium, direct pressure towards the table.

Right Sacral Base, direct pressure towards the table.

Left Sacral Base, direct pressure towards the table.

Right Sacral Apex, direct pressure towards the table.

Left Sacral Apex, direct pressure towards the table.

Right Ischium, hand cupping the base of the ischium and the pressure going headward.

Left Ischium, hand cupping the base of the ischium and the pressure going headward.

5th Lumbar spinous, thumb contact pressure towards the left.

5th Lumbar spinous, thumb contact pressure towards the right.

What have these tests told you?

1 and 3 look for Ilium AS (Gonstead).

2 and 4 look for Ilium PI.

5 and 6 look for a rotation of the Sacrum.

7 and 8 look for a rotation of the Sacral apex (this can move in relation to the base in the living Sacrum).

9 and 10 look for a slippage between the Ilia and the Sacrum.

11 and 12 look for spinous laterality of the 5th lumbar. Continue into the other lumbar vertebrae. To look for a straight posteriority, give a sharp pressure and release directly over the spinous, this will bounce the joint and a week arm indicates a posteriority.

Surrogate Testing

There are times when it not practical to test the patient. This may be because the patient is too young, too old or frail and not mentally competent. In this case, ask the caregiver to assist in the testing. Ask the caregiver to contact the patient whilst you test their arm and then go through the tests using the caregiver's arm as the test arm. Babies can be tested whilst lying on the mother's body, or held in her arms. You will be surprised just how accurate this method can be.

Testing And Amputee

If your patient only has one complete leg, how do you test for physiological short leg? Hold the good leg just below the knee and push headward (cephalic); test the arm. A weak arm means that the leg is short and you are increasing the shortness. Hold the leg just above the knee and press towards the foot (caudal) and test. A weakness would indicate and long leg.

APPENDIX LEGEND

APPENDIX	**A**	Category I Flow Chart
APPENDIX	**B**	SB PLUS & SB MINUS
APPENDIX	**C**	Occipital Line ONE
APPENDIX	**D**	Occipital Line TWO
APPENDIX	**E**	Occipital Line THREE
APPENDIX	**F**	CATEGORY II Flow Chart
APPENDIX	**G**	Trapezius Line
APPENDIX	**H**	CATEGORY III Flow Chart
APPENDIX	**I**	Dural Connections

CATEGORY I FLOW CHART

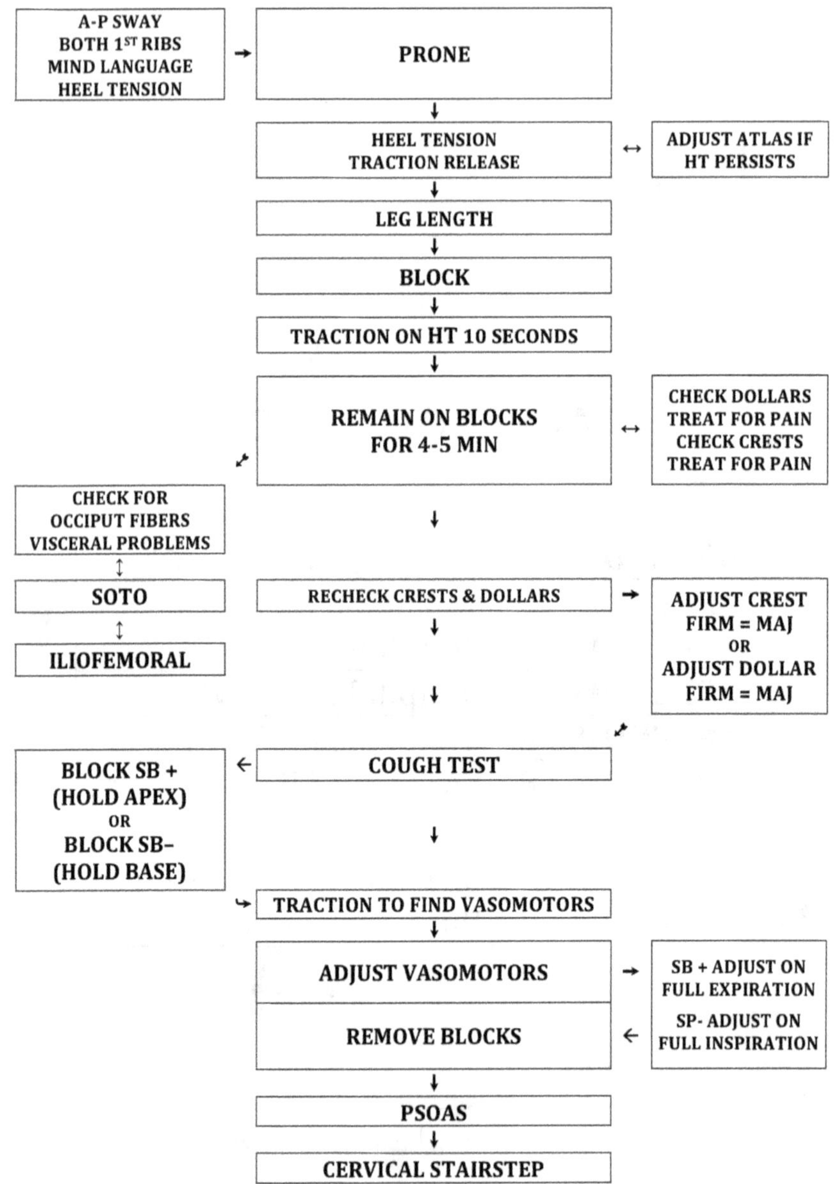

SB Plus SB Minus

If there was an SB + then the pressure is placed on the Apex of the Sacrum.

Adjust on full Inspiration as the patient inhales.

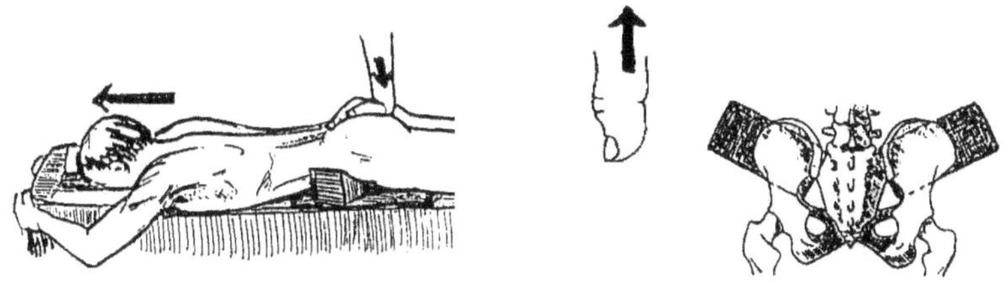

If there was an SB – then the pressure is placed on the Base of the Sacrum.

Adjust on full Expiration as the patient exhales.

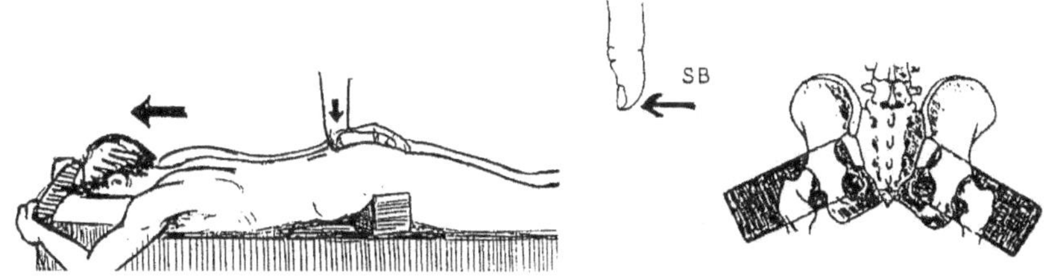

HOLD THE PRESSURE FOR FOUR SECONDS.

APPENDIX

OCCIPITAL LINE ONE

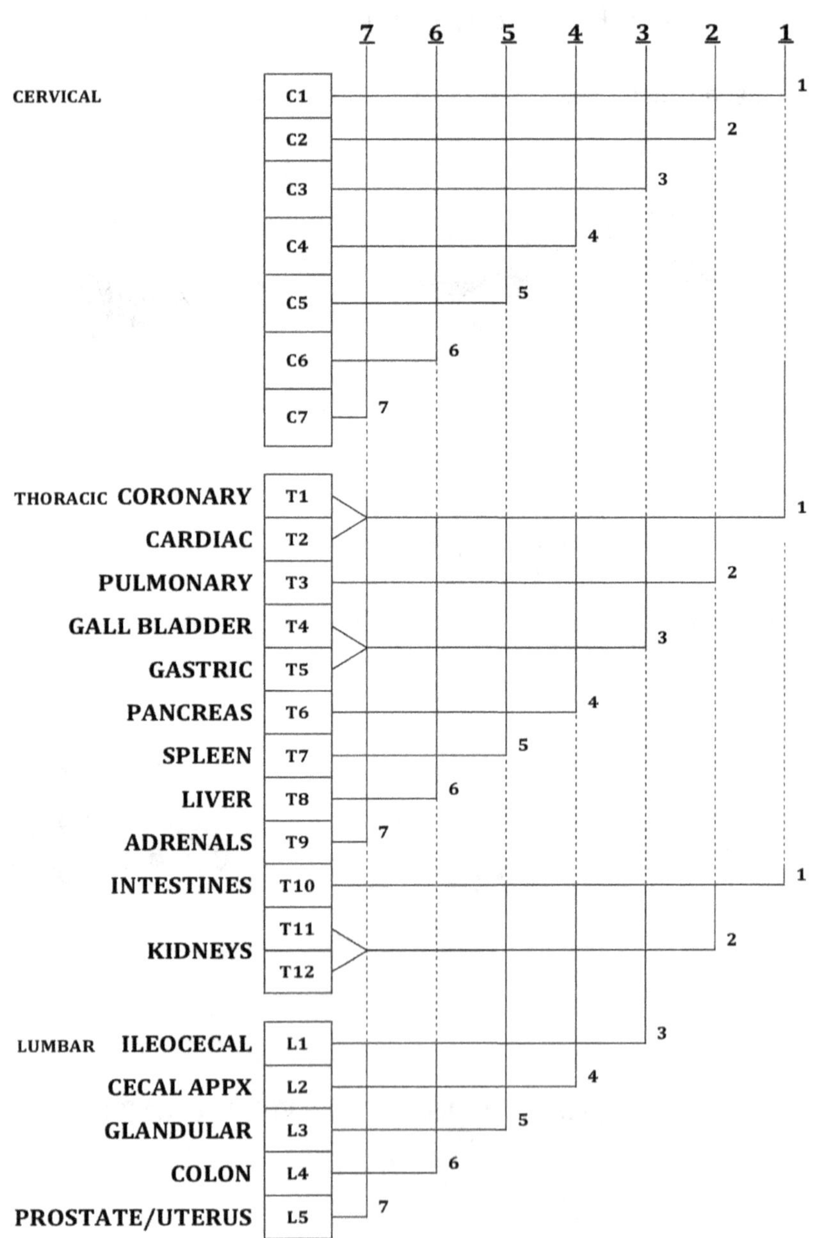

OCCIPITAL LINE TWO

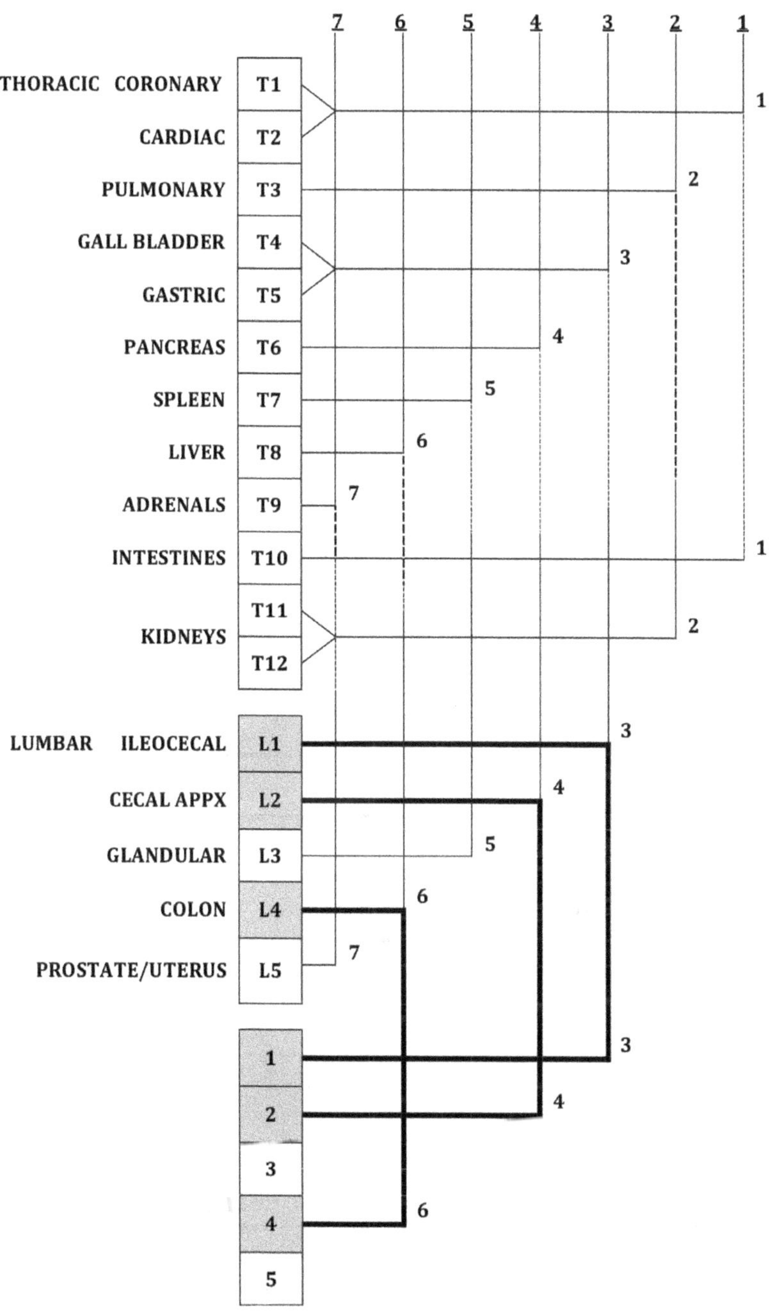

APPENDIX

OCCIPITAL LINE THREE

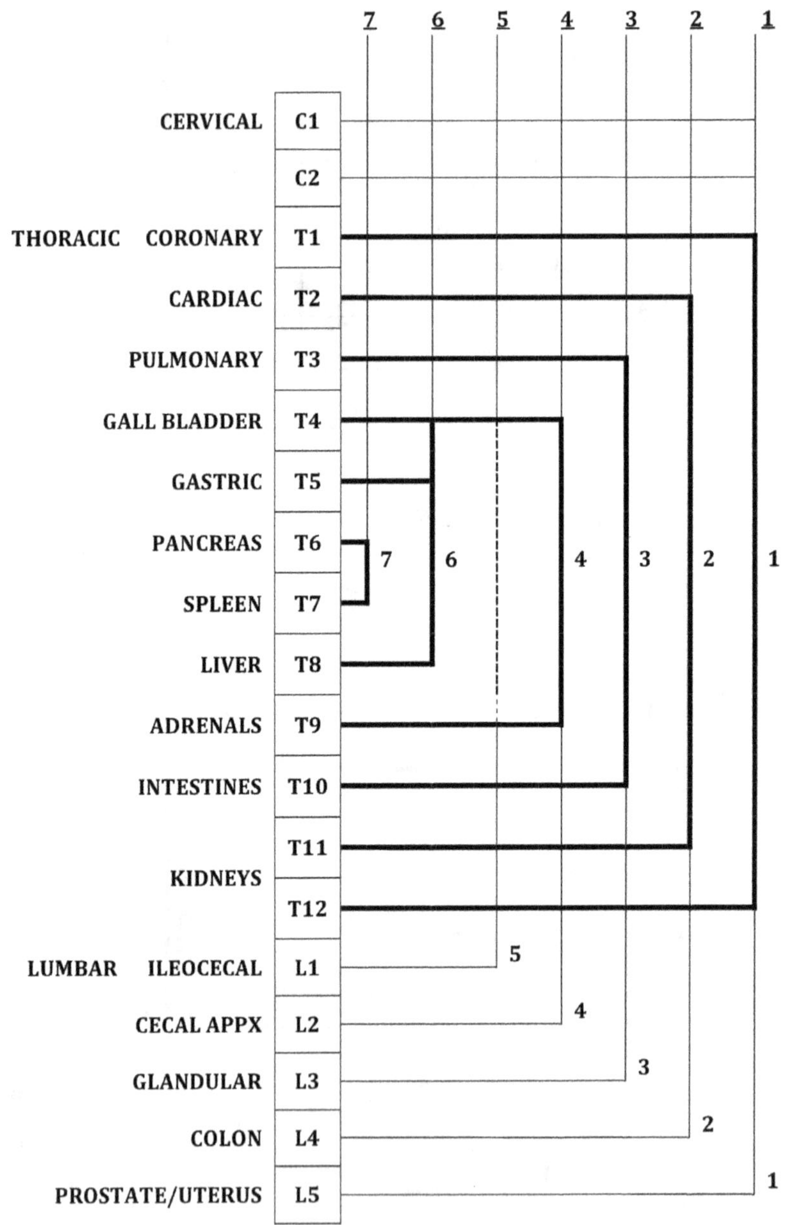

APPENDIX

CATEGORY II FLOW CHART

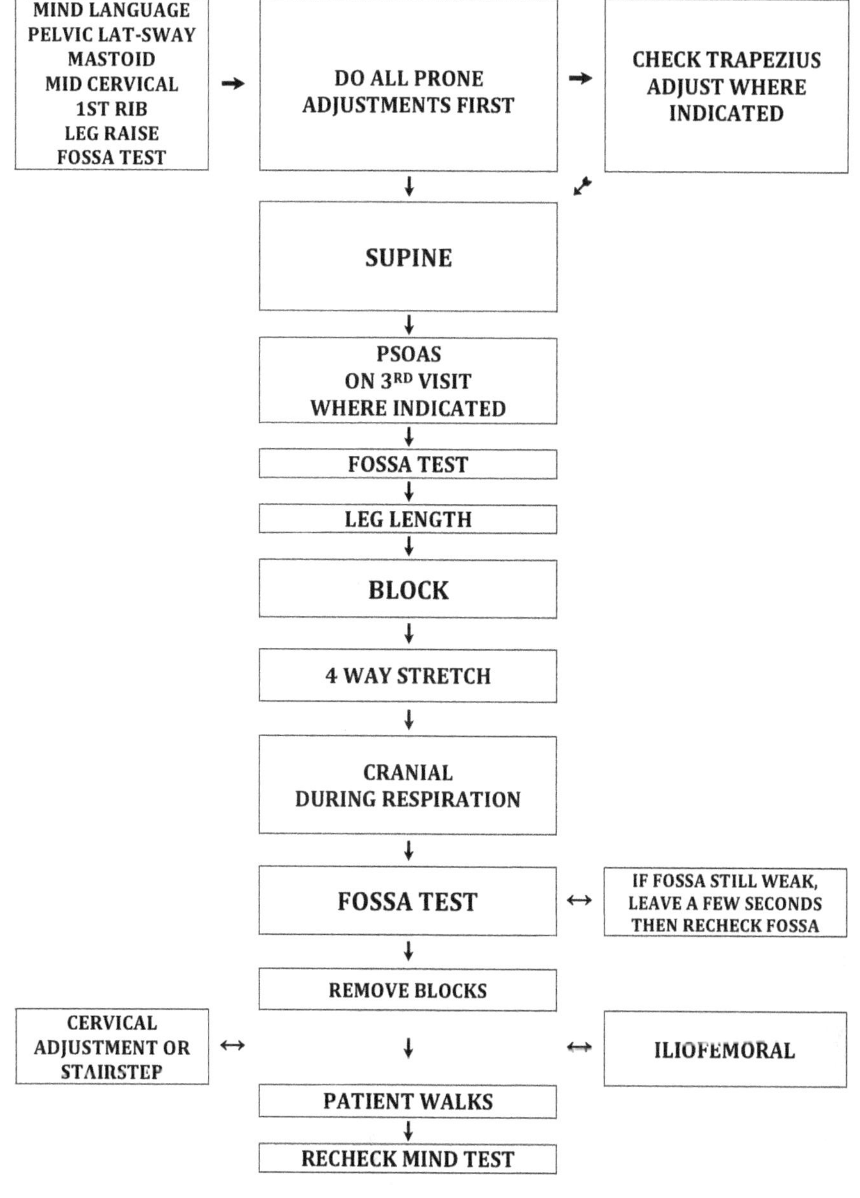

TRAPEZIUS ANALYTICAL CHARTS

Trapezius Line	7	6	5	4	3	2	1
Thoracic							
T1							1
T2							1
T3						2	
T4					3		
T5					3		
T6				4			
T7			5				
T8		6					
T9	7						
T10							1
T11						2	
T12						2	
Lumbar							
L1					3		
L2				4			
L3			5				
L4		6					
L5	7						

APPENDIX

CATEGORY III FLOW CHART

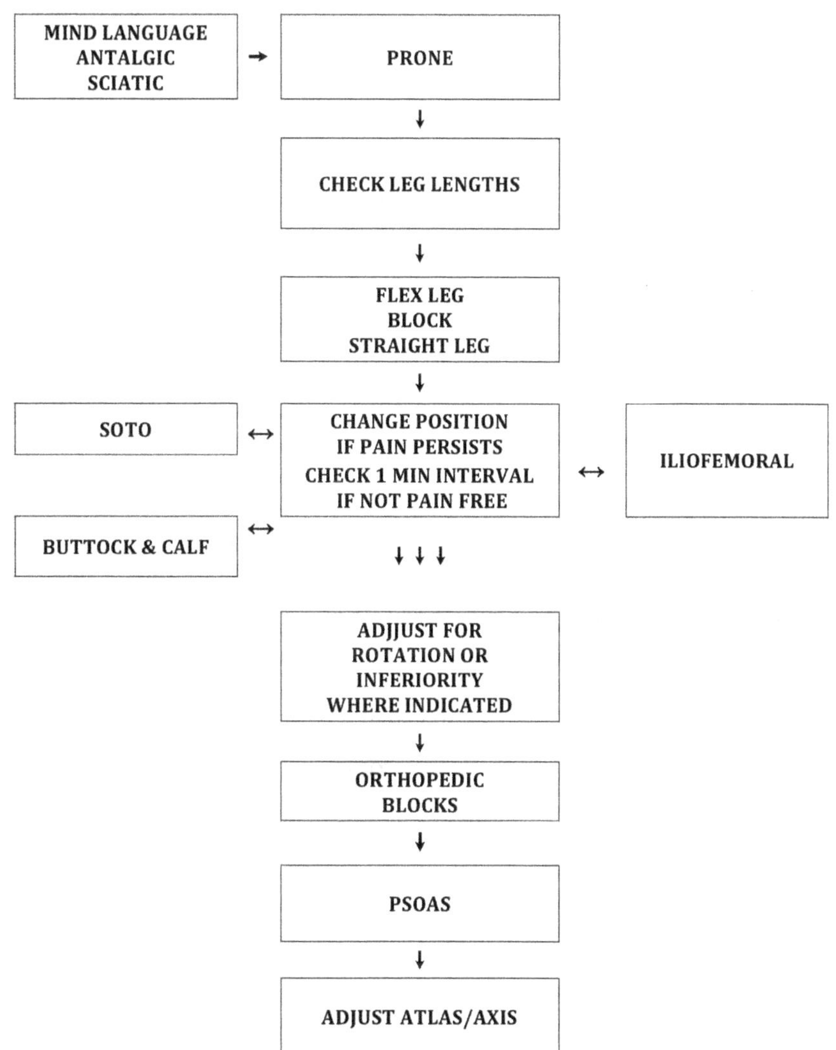

APPENDIX

Dural Connections

Contributed by Dr. Charles Blum

The issue of dural connections needs to be updated. Here is the way we understand it according the research.

It is not just about dural tensions but also about pia mater involvement:

The meningeal dura and periosteal dura in the cranium does have firm attachments to the internal periosteum of the cranium, and even passes through the sutures to have attachment into the external cranial periosteum. The dura then continues as a tube to attach firmly into the internal sacral canal in the region of the 2nd sacral segment.

From the external inward, there are various types of connections to the occiput, cervical, thoracic, lumbar and sacrum helping to maintain the dura and spinal cords optimal positioning during movement. These include the rectus capitus posterior minor [1], the ligamentum nuchae [2] and flava [3], the (thoracolumbar) ligaments of Hofman [4-6], and Trolards [6,7] (sacral) ligament.

The pia mater is a tissue that cannot be separated from the neural tissue without tearing that tissue. So, tensions to this tissue have a direct affect on neural tissue and are based upon, (1) the size of the brain relative to the foramen magnum and it not being able to be "pulled" downward through this canal, and (2) the firm attachment of the filum terminale at the coccyx [8]. Between each spinal nerve is a meningeal bridge of tissue that connects the dura mater to the pia mater called the dentate ligament.

Together with the dural attachments into the periosteum, the related myoligamentous connections for adjacent bones to the dura, the pia mater inherent tension due to the placement of the brain and filum terminale, and the dentate ligaments - these all create the patterns of tension that relate to the patterns of distortion found in SOT.

APPENDIX

References:

1. Hack GD, Koritzer RT, Robinson WL, Hallgren REC, Greenman PE. Anatomical relation between the rectus capitis posterior minor muscle and dura mater. *Spine,* Dec 1995; 20 (23): 2484-6.
2. Mitchell B, Humphreys BK, O'Sullivan E. Attachment of the ligamentum nuchae to cervical posterior spinal dura and the lateral part of the occipital bone, *Journal of Manipulative and Physiological Therapeutics.* Mar/Apr 1998; 21(3): 145-8.
3. Shinomiya K, Dawson J, Spengler DM, Konrad P, Blumenkopf. An analysis of the posterior epidural ligament role on the cervical spinal cord. *Spine,* Sep 1996. 21(18): 2081-8.
4. Bashline SD, Bilott JR, Ellis JP. Meningovertebral ligaments and their putative significance in low back pain. *Journal of Manipulative and Physiological Therapeutics.* Nov/Dec 1996; 19(9): 592-6.
5. Kershner DE, Binhammer RT. Lumbar intrathecal ligaments. *Clin Anat.* 2002 Mar; 15(2):82-7.
6. Scapinelli R. Anatomical and radiologic studies on the lumbosacral meningo-vertebral ligaments of humans. *J Spinal Disord.* Mar 1990; 3 (1): 6-15.
7. Barbaix E, Girardin MD, Hoppner JP, Van Roy P, Claris JP, Anterior sacrodural attachments Trolard's ligaments revisited Manual Therapy, Mar 2000; 1(2): 88-91.
8. Breig A. The biomechanics of the spinal cord and its membranes in the spinal canal. *Verh Anat Ges.* 1965; 115:49-69.

INDEX

INDEX

INDEX

I hope this book has sparked you interest in this fascinating approach to Chiropractic. I urge you to attend the seminars found in many states and countries around the world. Also, join the SOTO in your country. I am confident that once you have mastered the Sacro-Occipital Technique (SOT) you will never look back. Below are a few helpful links for reference.

Resourceful Links:

http://www.sotousa.com
http://www.soto.net.au
http://www.sorsi.com
http://www.sotoeurope.org

Bruce Vaughan DC, FICC
www.brucevaughan.com

INTERNATIONAL HEALTH PUBLISHING

Inspiring readers of the world to experience the light.
International Health Publishing books express truth and wisdom, encourage spiritual enlightenment, facilitate growth and healing – while also providing a phenomenal reading experience.

International Health Publishing's vision is to increase the number and quality of books and resources available to the public, students and Doctors of Chiropractic – allowing for greater understanding, increased education, as well as more visibility and accessibility of the Chiropractic profession as a means of preventative and continued health care.

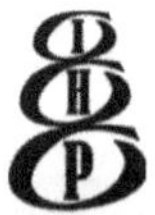

INTERNATIONAL HEALTH PUBLISHING
Adjusting and Growing
International Headquarters • Carrollton, Texas

www.InternationalHealthPublishing.com

www.ingramcontent.com/pod-product-compliance
Lightning Source LLC
Chambersburg PA
CBHW050524280326
41932CB00014B/2442

* 9 7 8 0 9 8 1 8 3 5 3 6 5 *